HEALTH PROMOTION PLANNING

HEALTH PROMOTION PLANNING

Learning from the Accounts of Public Health Practitioners

JEAN MARIE S. PLACE

JONEL THALLER

SCOTT S. HALL

JB JOSSEY-BASS™

A Wiley Brand

For general information on our other products and services or for technical support, please contact our Customer Care Department within the United States at (800) 762-2974, outside the United States at (317) 572-3993 or fax (317) 572-4002.

Wiley also publishes its books in a variety of electronic formats. Some content that appears in print may not be available in electronic formats. For more information about Wiley products, visit our web site at www.wiley.com.

Library of Congress Cataloging-in-Publication Data Applied for:

Paperback ISBN: 9781119686187

Cover Design: Wiley
Cover Image: © Thomas H. Mitchell/500px/Getty Images

Set in 10.5/12.5pt TimesLTStd by Straive, Pondicherry, India

To my mentors, for introducing me to
a profession I am passionate about.
To my Muncie community, for teaching me.
To Obed, Allie, and Ava, for your
incredible love.

Jean Marie S. Place

CONTENTS

NOTE TO INSTRUCTORS

This book includes multiple stories of how a community addresses the opioid crisis. The stories are based on interviews that we, the authors, conducted. We spoke with many public health practitioners, seeking to learn more about the programs they manage, wanting to understand how these programs work to mitigate the opioid epidemic. We include true stories in this book for the purpose of providing instructional examples, but we do not reveal the county where this work takes place, and we use pseudonyms to protect the practitioners who shared their stories with us. In some stories, small elements in the storyline or sequencing of events have been fictionalized.

In this book, we approach program planning through the lens of a specific health problem so that students can see how multiple programs work together to affect a public health issue. Although we recognize that many public health issues are interconnected, we chose to take a closer look at substance use – and specifically opioid use disorder – to explore how public health practitioners are implementing programs to address this devastating social problem. The opioid crisis is an especially salient societal challenge of which students and instructors are likely to have some basic knowledge or interest. Considering the wide range of this issue, they may even have a personal connection. Consequently, we chose to highlight key principles of program planning by describing programmatic efforts related to addressing substance use and opioid-related problems. In this way, students can learn more about program planning while, at the same time, learning more about substance use.

Our emphasis on the real-life accounts of public health professionals is intended to help students see and discuss program planning principles in action. As you will see, public health professionals can include social workers, case managers, therapists, program evaluators, program administrators, and medical specialists, among others. Ultimately, we want students to feel like the people they meet in this text are relatable and the projects they discuss are achievable, thus furthering an investment in becoming public health professionals themselves. We hope, foremost, that students come away with a better understanding of the principles and processes of building health promotion programs, especially for substance use prevention, treatment, and recovery. A deeper knowledge of the opioid epidemic is an added, beneficial outcome.

This textbook does not necessarily depict comprehensive program planning, nor does it detail in-depth explanations of the opioid epidemic, but it does provide honest, real-world information from the frontlines to help bring these topics to life. You might find it useful to supplement its content with select articles or other textbooks such as Green and Kreuter's (2005) *Health Program Planning: An Educational and Ecological Approach* or McKenzie, Neiger, and Thackeray's (2017) *Planning, Implementing, and Evaluating Health Promotion Programs*. In our book, program planning concepts emerge in the course of accounts – or stories – revolving around a person or organization in a given context; the information is driven primarily by the organizations and events we were able to witness and investigate further and, thus, they may lack some elements of inclusivity.

Each chapter will end with discussion questions and activities that can be used by an instructor to spark conversations among students about principles of health promotion planning. These resources can also be used as individual or group assignments, as adapted by instructors. We hope that you will find these tools helpful as you embark on your learning journey.

FOREWORD

Prescription painkillers – ostensibly harmless, even helpful, tablets offered by physicians and stored in medicine cabinets above our bathroom sinks – hit our unsuspecting synapses with the pleasure-packed thrill of leaping out of an airplane. Many intravenous heroin users can trace their addiction back to misusing painkillers, in some cases legitimately prescribed. These pills, and their opioid-derived counterparts such as heroin, fentanyl, and carfentanyl, kill approximately 130 Americans per day, driving down our nation's average life expectancy and mercilessly bringing people who were previously at the prime of their lives into an early grave.

The undergraduate students I teach in my public health course knew nothing about these statistics. Many were not familiar with the word "opioid," although Schedule II narcotics are responsible for the biggest public health crisis of our time. It was staggering to realize that what my students knew about opioids might be limited to Percocet prescriptions for wisdom teeth or a handful of pills pharmed out at parties.

As I came into my own awareness of this community crisis, I did an about-face in my syllabus design, reexamining whether definition-heavy textbooks with piecemeal examples from a range of A to Z topics were packing the punch necessary to help students learn about the public health issues that plague us. As an experiment, I tried teaching a semester-long, health promotion planning course through an in-depth examination of *one* relevant, pressing area – opioid misuse. Didactically, the question was whether a high-resolution lens focused intensely on one issue could reveal more to my students about public health principles than a series of quick, cursory glances across the landscape.

In this class, we turned the camera to opioids. The master syllabus remained the same – I still had to teach about the major components of planning, implementing, and evaluating health promotion programs – but as we zeroed in on the opioid epidemic, paradoxically, we began to see a more panoramic view. We talked details about medication-assisted treatment (MAT), post-incarceration support, prescription monitoring, syringe exchanges, and supervised consumption spaces. Like individual trees in the proverbial forest, these successful health promotion programs marked the path to a vista where we could see a wide-angle view. We talked more broadly about concepts like health promotion planning models, theories, and strategies. These concepts emerged organically and in context, tied as they were to the programs we discussed. My students began to see the myriad of ways that public health concepts interact when mitigating a specific threat to public health. They saw the forest for the trees.

That semester my students and I walked away with a bargain. We understood the principles and processes of building health promotion programs *and* had a deeper knowledge of the opioid epidemic. I knew I wanted to teach this way again. I began envisioning a book that could accompany this "high resolution" way of teaching. It should provide definitions and descriptions of program planning, but also anchor them to one specific public health topic and embed them in a story.

The vision has come to fruition in this collection of accounts – or real-world stories of public health professionals. Our goal is to facilitate practical understanding and application of these concepts by sharing stories of real people in a real community using concepts and models from health promotion planning. Our job was to draw lessons from what our local public health practitioners shared with us, pointing out the principles of health promotion planning behind the outcomes. We hope that familiar people, places, and events will come to mind as you read these stories, providing a visual illustration of concepts that we sometimes only talk about in a detached and overly simplistic way. We hope this book will be beneficial to instructors and students because it is both readable and relevant.

Thank you for joining us in this journey,

Jean Marie S. Place, PhD, MPH, MSW
June 22, 2023

ACKNOWLEDGMENTS

We want to thank the many public health practitioners who shared their stories with us, invited us into their organizations, and revealed the ups and downs of program planning. Thank you!

INTRODUCTION

WHY TALK ABOUT SUBSTANCE USE?

Before you begin this section, ask yourself if you believe substance misuse is a public health problem. If you affirmed that substance misuse is a public health problem, can you describe why you believe so? In this introduction, we want to encourage you to think broadly about substance misuse – specifically opioid misuse – and how it has affected individuals, families, and communities. Consider how program planning principles can help public health practitioners address serious issues, such as the opioid epidemic.

Substance misuse (including addiction) is one of the major health challenges of our day. Societal-wide problems have accelerated swiftly and savagely – the result of a storm of social, economic, and political forces that contributed to the easy availability of opioids and other illicit substances in the United States. Public health professionals have spent countless hours planning and implementing programs to battle the effects of this major challenge.

How big of a problem are we talking about? In 2022, nearly 110,000 American lives were lost to drug overdose. Drug deaths had steadily increased over 2020 and 2021, with a 17% and 30% increase, respectively (Centers for Disease Control [CDC], 2023). Most of these deaths are attributed to opioids (Scholl et al., 2019), with synthetic opioids like fentanyl contributing to roughly 75% of the deaths. On any given day, roughly 130 Americans die because of the misuse of an opioid (National Center for Drug Abuse Statistics, 2023).[1]

The US Department of Health and Human Services declared a national public health emergency in 2017 due to unprecedented,

---

[1] There is a difference between "opioid" and "opiate." An opiate is all natural, coming from the poppy plant (opium, codeine, morphine) with an analgesic effect, meaning it relieves pain. An opioid is synthetic or partly synthetic. The term opioid is often used to refer to both natural and synthetic forms because many natural forms of the molecule will go through a synthetic process before hitting the market. For example, heroin uses opium molecules but is created synthetically.

Health Promotion Planning: Learning from the Accounts of Public Health Practitioners, First Edition. Jean Marie S. Place, Jonel Thaller, and Scott S. Hall.
© 2024 John Wiley & Sons, Inc. Published 2024 by John Wiley & Sons, Inc.

nationwide opioid abuse. Former director of the Centers for Disease Control Robert Redfield called it "the public health issue of our time." What does that mean for you as an aspiring professional? How might the challenges of addiction affect those you interact with in your career? How might your career be shaped by the challenging, urgent threat of substance misuse, specifically opioid misuse, even if you do not directly work with a population that uses these substances?

Before we discuss the wide array of programmatic efforts aimed at addressing something like opioid misuse, we want to provide context on opioids to firmly establish the substance use epidemic as a matter of public health. The information provided below is intended to make clear how the opioid epidemic affects the public, and why students who are trained to develop prevention and treatment programs for an individual, family, or community unit are a vital workforce. Take a look at this brief overview on how opioid use disorder (OUD) fits the criteria for being a public health problem.

IS THE PROBLEM PREVENTABLE?

- Substance misuse, including misuse of opioids, is a preventable problem. Much of what puts people at risk for substance misuse can be minimized – and efforts to prevent opioid misuse and overdose can save and improve many lives. For example, the CDC (2021) offered several methods for reducing opioid overdose deaths. First, medical professionals can improve how and when opioids are prescribed to patients. Overall exposure to opioids can be reduced when medical professionals and other practitioners promote alternative pain treatment, including emotional and cognitive pain management skills. Further, education and public awareness of opioid misuse and its consequences can be improved and expanded, and best practices of treating those with OUD can be made more abundant and accessible. Other approaches may become more apparent as you continue reading about the causes and effects of opioid-related problems.

WHAT IS THE MAGNITUDE OF THE PROBLEM?

- As is apparent in the statistics already mentioned, the magnitude of substance-misuse-related deaths is staggering. Furthermore, upwards of 930,000 people in the United States died of a drug overdose from 1999 to 2020, with opioid-related deaths increasing more than eight times in the past two decades (National Center for Health Statistics, 2021). More than two out of every three drug overdoses involve opioids (Hedegaard et al., 2021). Aside from overdoses, close to one million people received medication-assisted treatments to manage their OUD in the past year (Substance Abuse and Mental Health Services Administration [SAMHSA], 2022). Moreover, nearly 5 million individuals ages 12 and older reported having misused prescription pain relievers (SAMHSA, 2022). Consider how many lives are affected by this problem when including those who love, care for, and depend on people struggling with substance use disorder.

■ The opioid misuse problem has gotten worse over time. While data from 2022 suggests that a staggering increase in overdose deaths has begun to level off, in earlier years the United States faced an astronomic rise in such deaths. From 2019 to 2020, there was an age-adjusted 31% increase in overdose deaths, with some states seeing upwards of a 50% increase in overdose deaths within one year (CDC, 2021). From 2013 to 2017, the average annual increase of drug overdose deaths due to synthetic opioids was 75% per year, slowing but still increasing 9% per year from 2017 through 2019 (Hedegaard et al., 2020). In recent years, opioids accounted for over 68,000 deaths in 2020 – a dramatic increase from just under 48,000 such deaths in 2017 (CDC, 2022).

WHAT ARE THE COSTS ASSOCIATED WITH THE PROBLEM?

■ Financially, the total economic burden of the opioid epidemic in the United States is estimated to be about $1,021 billion each year, including costs of OUD at $471 billion and costs associated with fatal opioid overdose estimated at $550 billion (Luo et al., 2021). This economic burden includes costs from healthcare, lost productivity, addiction treatment, and criminal justice involvement. On the flipside, for every person that does not develop an OUD, significant financial value is generated. For every person that does not develop an OUD, $2.2 million is generated from a societal perspective, $325,125 from a taxpayer perspective, and $244,030 from a healthcare sector perspective (Murphy, 2021).

■ Other costs of opioid-related problems are more physical in nature. For example, infants born with opioids in their blood suffer withdrawal from the dissipation of the substance, known as neonatal abstinence syndrome (Hirai et al., 2021). Opioid misuse can also contribute to the spread of infectious diseases like HIV and Hepatitis C through contaminated needles used to inject the substance (CDC, 2021). Incarceration rates also increase with greater misuse of opioids, separating those who struggle with OUD even farther from much-needed prosocial interaction and support (Scott et al., 2021).

Estimates suggest that OUD has cost US taxpayers around $93 billion. Such costs include nearly $30 billion for criminal justice system expenses and $63 billion in excessive healthcare expenses. The additional loss of productivity in the workforce due to premature deaths is estimated to be about $65 billion (Murphy, 2021).

This sampling of facts and figures begins to give us an idea of how OUD is considered a public health problem. Finding solutions to this problem can be especially difficult. By the time a person reaches a state of active opioid addiction they have, by definition, become dependent on the substance and can experience extremely painful, and sometimes dangerous, withdrawal symptoms if they quit using. Moreover, in active addiction, the brain has developed an increased tolerance to the drug, needing a progressively higher dose of it to avoid these withdrawal symptoms. Many public health professionals push for preventing misuse before it starts, for example, by working to help people avoid adverse childhood experiences (ACEs) that tend to predict substance use in later life (Leza et al., 2021; Rogers et al., 2022).

Despite the overwhelming nature of this work, addressing public health problems like opioid misuse is essential for the welfare of society. As you will see in the next section, families can play a major role in substance-related problems. We suspect that many people can relate in some way to the positive and negative impact families can have on an individual's growth and development, and we invite you to consider the importance of incorporating families into planning and implementing solutions to public health problems.

We will now take a deeper dive into how OUD creates a burden for families.

WHAT DO WE KNOW ABOUT OPIOIDS AND FAMILIES?

Many of us love someone, or know someone who loves someone, who is struggling with addiction. So powerful is the pull of addiction that our loved ones often become unrecognizable to us. In recent years, over 500,000 children were living with an adult with OUD, an increase of 30% since 2002 (Bullinger & Wing, 2019). Children raised in homes with drug abuse are at elevated risks for neglect, abuse, unsanitary living conditions, witnessing domestic violence, and having limited resources (Barnard & McKeganey, 2004; Taplin & Mattick, 2015). Studies show that children who live in a home where there is opioid misuse generally experience psychological distress and reduced family cohesion (Ashrafioun et al., 2011). Adults who misuse opioids often report that they were mistreated as children, and research suggests that opioids are preferred by such adults due to the numbing effects of the substance (Maté, 2010). Opioid prescriptions given to family members increase the likelihood that individuals without opioid prescriptions overdose on opioids, meaning family members can be a key source of access to opioids (Khan et al., 2019).

Parents who have substance use disorder may adversely impact their children in a variety of ways, not withstanding the love they have for their children. Opioid use during pregnancy increases the risk of fetal underdevelopment and babies born suffering from withdrawal symptoms, such as tremors, poor sleep, irritability, and feeding difficulties (Schiff & Patrick, 2017; Wexelblatt et al., 2018). Moreover, sometimes pregnant women with an OUD avoid proper prenatal care due to stigma or fear of child protective services involvement (Schempf & Strobino, 2009). Infants and toddlers may struggle to form healthy attachments to parents who are in active addiction and struggling with OUD, which makes children more vulnerable to stress and emotion dysregulation (Cook et al., 2017).

Parents with OUD can become preoccupied with drug seeking and may engage less often with their young children (Young & Martin, 2012). Opioid dependence can alter a parent's brain, replacing the natural pleasure-inducing experience of relationships with drug cravings (Mitsi & Zachariou, 2016). As children age, they continue to be at risk for inadequate parenting. Parents who struggle with OUD frequently engage in more negative parenting behaviors and fewer positive parenting behaviors (Peisch et al., 2018). They have also been found to use harsher and more humiliating punishment (Peisch et al., 2018).

In general, parental substance misuse contributes to less parental monitoring and supervision and less parental warmth and support, putting children of any age at risk for developmental and behavioral problems (Barnes et al., 2000). Children are also at risk for becoming parentified – meaning, they are expected to take on the role of a caregiver to a needy parent, which puts excessive pressure on children to behave beyond their capacities (Godsall et al., 2004). Ultimately, parents with OUD are at risk of losing their children to the foster care system, and research suggests that children remain in the system longer and are less likely to be reunited with their parents when opioids are involved, compared to other substances (Grella et al., 2009; Mirick & Steenrod, 2016). This may be due to such mothers having a stronger addiction and especially low financial and housing stability (Grella et al., 2009). Moreover, parents who lose custody of their children are less likely to recover from OUD (Comiskey, 2013).

In some families, children are the opioid users. In recent years, between roughly 12% and 14% of high schoolers in the United States admitted to having misused prescription opioids in the past (CDC, 2021). Adolescents are at risk for poorer judgment due to the neurological gap between their expanding reward system and slowly developing cognitive control functions (Chassin et al., 2013), which can contribute to substance misuse. Furthermore, living in a rural setting seems to correspond with higher adolescent opioid misuse by as much as 35% (Monnat & Rigg, 2016), and adolescent opioid use is strongly linked to depression (Edlunda et al., 2015). Dealing with adolescent substance misuse can be overbearing for parents, some of whom may cope by turning to substances themselves, which in turn can escalate the risks for poorer parenting and subsequent child outcomes (Leonard & Eiden, 2007).

As noted earlier, family dynamics often play key roles in opioid misuse problems. They can also be a contributing factor to other public health challenges and outcomes. Multiple theoretical perspectives help us understand why families and other social contexts can have such a powerful influence on problematic behaviors and societal trends. These perspectives are important to consider when addressing various public health problems.

HOW DO SOCIAL CONTEXTS INFLUENCE PROBLEMATIC BEHAVIOR SUCH AS SUBSTANCE MISUSE?

Public health initiatives hinge on the assumption that people have the capacity to change their behavior and health status. Yet, changing deeply engrained habits of thinking and doing can be extremely difficult – especially when the *social environment*, or the life circumstances and social interactions that surround and envelope a person, does not support the change.

Systems theory helps us visualize how the social environment influences human behavior. Through this lens, we see that individuals (and groups of individuals) operate as wholly functioning systems that are likewise comprised of functional subsystems. A family system, for example, can contain unique sibling-to-sibling or parent-to-child subsystems, each with its own dynamic and history.

Systems are functional in that each individual part contributes to the whole in a generally predictable manner. Individual family members often assume, whether consciously or not, a distinct role within the system, such as that of protector, caretaker, scapegoat, cheerleader, or peacekeeper. But, having specific roles does not imply that a system is necessarily promoting health and wellbeing or encouraging an ideal distribution of power among members. Some family systems can be highly dysfunctional, even for long spans of time. While internal or external forces can significantly disrupt a system and warrant a temporary adjustment, the system will naturally seek a return to *homeostasis*, or its previous state of operation.

Conceptualizing family systems in this way helps to understand why some people continue problematic behavior even when they express a desire to change it. Consider people who say they want to quit misusing drugs because of health issues but have been raised in a family where substance use is encouraged as part of leisure and bonding. Or, consider a person with a substance use disorder who have family members who thrive in caring for and rescuing the individual from their self-inflicted consequences. For these people, the decision to cease substance misuse, a positive behavior change, impacts the regular functioning of the system by disrupting routine interactions and altering assigned roles. Thus, behavior change is not as simple as one person changing their behavior. The context of their social environment must be taken into consideration.

Urie Bronfenbrenner's (1979) **ecological systems theory**[2] expands the family systems framework by incorporating an ecological perspective, taking into account multiple layers of influence from the social environment. This theory incorporates multiple layers of external systemic influences: the micro-, mezzo- (or exo-), and macrosystems. Another level of influence, the mesosystem, recognizes interactions that occur between systems at the mezzo-/exo-level. Moreover, the chronosystem refers to the influence of time and human development, such as adolescence, on human behavior.

The *microsystem* is comprised of all of an individual's personal characteristics and personality traits, including health and mental health conditions, strengths, challenges, and goals. A person who is struggling with addiction may be also grappling with severe anxiety or depression. They may have experienced sudden abandonment or a painful injury at some point in their life history. They may be young or old, raised in affluence or generational poverty. They may be highly educated or may have dropped out of high school. They may have a genetic disposition to addiction. All of these factors influence their behavior and belief in what is wise and possible.

The *mezzosystem*, also sometimes referred to as the *exo-system*, refers to the small groups, communities, or organizations to which an individual belongs, such as their family, school, neighborhood, workplace, or recreational groups. As with the microsystem, interactions within the mezzosystem can have a significant effect on a person's capacity for behavior change and ability to thrive. Peer and family systems have a huge impact on individual success in recovery from a substance use disorder. Human beings naturally long to connect with others, and group membership is a crucial component

---

[2] The ecological systems theory is also referred to as ecosystems theory, bioecological theory, or the socio-ecological model.

in identity development and maintenance of self-concept. In the addiction recovery community, the phrase "people, places, and things" is often used to refer to components of a person's environment that can trigger a return to substance misuse. Some connections provide easy access to substances and normalize their misuse.

The *macrosystem* refers to influence on human behavior at a societal and cultural level. Powerful institutions, such as the criminal justice system, the healthcare system, government, the media, and religion all impact opportunities and norms and trickle down into the decisions people make about their lives. For example, institutional biases against people with addictions, criminalization of certain substances but not others, representations of substance misuse portrayed by the media, and common constructions of race, class, and gender influence public perceptions of substance use. The influence of these macro-factors may sometimes be difficult for an individual to perceive directly but are nonetheless significant enough to influence behavior.

Any of these systems can be targeted when planning a behavior change strategy. For example, social workers work with individuals and families, but also within larger systems, such as neighborhoods and organizations, to facilitate improvements in health and wellbeing. At a macro-level, family policy experts advocate for policy change by working closely with legislative bodies. Likewise, public health workers engage in health education that can occur on a micro-level, with an individual, or on a macro-level if the goal is to bring about a culture change, establishing new behavioral norms.

External influences of human behavior can also be categorized as social, economic, and political forces. **Social forces** (Cox, 1981; Callero, 2017) are the core values and beliefs generally in a person's social environment, determining what behavior is normal and what is taboo, such as whether it is acceptable to use illegal drugs as a leisure activity. **Economic forces** (Heilbroner & Thurow, 1998; Estola, 2001) determine the availability of resources to individuals and communities, and whether people have access to the resources they need to merely survive or, conversely, whether their access to money, material goods, and special services might enable them to thrive. **Political forces** (Elkins, 1979; Gonidec, 1981) refer to the distribution of power or, more specifically, who makes the laws and what activities are considered criminal. These forces often work together to shape perceptions and responses to public health concerns. For example, we saw all of these forces converge with the increase in federal funding to support expansion of substance misuse treatment once the problem began to affect a more affluent demographic of users (Hoagland et al., 2019).

Social, economic, and political forces can also be considered **social determinants of health** – significant factors within the social environment that impact health and wellbeing, as well as overall functioning and quality of life.

Understanding the scope of a public health problem (e.g. the extents of opioid misuse and overdoses) and the roles played by social contexts (e.g. family, economy, culture) that encourage or maintain problematic behaviors help set the stage for addressing the problem. Effective prevention and intervention efforts require significant preparation and planning. Premature implementation of intended solutions can lead to a waste of opportunities and resources and could even make problems worse.

HOW CAN PROGRAM PLANNING HELP SOLVE PUBLIC HEALTH PROBLEMS?

A **program** is a set of activities organized toward a specific goal, and that goal typically involves influencing human behavior in some manner. Health promotion and social service programs are intended to improve the quality of life for individuals, families, and/or communities, building upon capacity and strengths that are already present to increase positive outcomes and reduce negative ones. In many ways, program planning and implementation is a form of carefully orchestrated problem solving, and it begins with a clear need or problem that should be addressed.

As you will see throughout this book, program planning is foundational to addressing public health problems, including opioid misuse. Public health professionals should be aware of various considerations in their planning efforts. Successful programs often target multiple factors that simultaneously contribute to a given problem. Such a complex approach requires careful, intentional planning. Given our focus on opioid misuse, and the relevance of familial factors for many individuals who struggle with this problem, especially minors, we now provide examples of how program planning can incorporate family-oriented elements in efforts to address the opioid epidemic.

In the case of opioid misuse prevention efforts, programs that target children should consider involving their parents. Clearly parents have a major influence on their children's drug-related decisions and behaviors, and the family environment overall can provide risk and protective factors that predict children's substance use (Swadi, 1999). Parents also influence children's attitudes about substances, with more favorable attitudes predicting future substance use (Guo et al., 2001; Messler et al., 2014). Prevention efforts can include educating parents about addiction and opioid misuse and how to reduce the risk of their children getting involved with substance misuse (US Department of Justice – Drug

Enforcement Administration & US Department of Education – Office of Safe & Healthy Students, 2017). Parents can help by teaching children healthy coping behaviors and using healthy parenting practices in general (Henderson et al., 2009). Efforts to prevent opioid misuse among parents should also account for the likelihood that such parents also often struggle with depression and anxiety (Martins et al., 2009), face social isolation from the community (Suchman et al., 2006), and may live in high-conflict and low-support home environments (Spehr et al., 2017). Helping parents who are dealing with grief, loss, and past or current trauma can decrease the likelihood that they turn to substances (Garrett & Landau, 2007).

Program planning often also means preparing intervention efforts that help individuals and families end and recover from opioid misuse. Successful family-based treatment strategies typically combine home visits with counseling (Barnard & McKeganey, 2004; O'Farrell & Clements, 2012). Planning related to treatment and intervention benefits from a comprehensive, ecological approach that addresses family dynamics and other systems outside of the home, such as schools, aftercare services, community policies, and cultural norms and behaviors (Fischer & Lyness, 2005). Seeking commitments from schools, communities, and leaders to support children and families is critical for wide ranging success (Boyd & Faden, 2002).

When programming focuses on parents' opioid misuse, program developers should consider the various ways that children fit into the circumstances. For example, some parents avoid seeking treatment because of a lack of childcare options, though having children can also motivate parents to recover from substance misuse (Taplin & Mattick, 2015). Children need help coping with a parent with an OUD and may need a more stable place to live for a time. Even though parental recovery from substance abuse is a positive outcome, it can also be an especially stressful time for the family. Familiar family patterns and routines get disrupted, making the recovery period potentially more challenging for children than before recovery, even if ultimately the family environment improves (Lewis & Allen-Byrd, 2007). Program planning should account for additional stress during the early recovery period and help ensure that new family patterns form that help prevent relapse and other risk factors that could contribute to children's substance misuse.

Considering all the influences that may lead a person to misuse opioids for the first, second, and subsequent times, prevention and intervention efforts must cast a wide net. Broadly, problematic human behavior and social trends are complex and often require complex solutions. Throughout this book, we provide a variety of examples of public health professionals working hard to address opioid-related problems. Such efforts are built from a foundation of program planning and their stories allow a glimpse into important planning processes. These are real-life examples that typically illustrate a mixture of both ideal and less-than-ideal procedures, creating opportunities to critically evaluate lessons that can be applied in the future. In practice, our best intentions do not always translate into the implementation of best practices, but being able to adapt to novel circumstances is also an essential part of program planning.

HOW WILL THIS BOOK BE STRUCTURED?

The content in this book is delivered through professionals' own accounts of their public health work. We conducted formal and informal interviews with more than 100 people who live and work in a small midwestern city with an *Americana* feel. In tandem with the interviews, we observed coalition meetings in action, took notes at townhalls, ate with people in active addiction at community-centered meals, and visited extensively with public health professionals, clinicians, social workers, and elected officials trying to find solutions to an ever-increasing crisis.

The people named in each of the accounts are real people with fictional names used to mask their identities. Embedded within these stories are key insights into program planning. We have highlighted insights that can serve as stepping stones for each of us as we advance public health practice in our own communities. Interventions should be built on a solid foundation of knowledge, expertise, and evidence, and so we have tried to point out public health principles as they are revealed in the context of a story.

Finally, we provide discussion questions to consider at the end of the chapter. Use these to further reflect on what can be learned and adapted from these professional accounts and applied to other communities.

Please know that our intent is not to provide an exhaustive list of interventions used to address the opioid epidemic. Rather, the chapters in this textbook describe the tools used by one community at one point in time. In this way, the stories are limited in scope and cannot underscore every important learning principle. Nevertheless, we hope readers get a feel for how public health practice is implemented in communities across the United States – imperfect and imprecise, but full of lessons for future generations to absorb as they take up the torch in addressing a devastating national crisis.

CHAPTER GUIDE

- In Chapter 1, we introduce Flynn Mosi who is in charge of a community-wide needs assessment. Use this chapter to learn more about the basics of conducting large-scale needs assessments. We illuminate the difference between primary and secondary data, identify different sources for data collection, and discuss how needs are prioritized for intervention.

- In Chapter 2, we introduce Fabiola Martin who engages her team in another type of needs assessment, a fatality review board. They look at the untimely deaths of people lost to substance misuse and seek to learn lessons from these deaths to better help those who struggle with OUD. Use this chapter to understand risk factors and levels of prevention.
- In Chapter 3, we describe a maternal treatment center for women with OUD during pregnancy and in the postpartum period. We introduce a staff member named Kate who wants to help the women but does not have a complete understanding of the barriers women face in treatment. She works with staff to improve their program based on the results of a consumer analysis conducted among women with substance use disorder, particularly OUD. Use this chapter to get a better understanding of the socio-ecological model and barriers and facilitators that affect health outcomes. We also discuss qualitative and quantitative research in a community setting, and how research results can inform program planning.
- In Chapter 4, we introduce Juli Kohl who organizes an event to celebrate recovery from substance use disorders. We explore the logistics of event planning, including forming a planning committee, developing financial sources of support, marketing to vendors and participants, and evaluating an event's success. Use this chapter to learn about implementation management.
- In Chapter 5, we introduce Darby Montegro who brings a prevention program to schools and an awareness event to the community. In this chapter, we focus on understanding a theoretical model for behavior change, as well as implementation considerations like obtaining sources of support.
- In Chapter 6, we introduce Fanny Brown, the facilitator of a health education program who faces challenges in participant recruitment. We discuss social marketing principles that can be leveraged to address recruitment concerns. We also review the evaluation of health education programs and discuss the importance of having a strong evidence base to support continued implementation.
- In Chapter 7, we introduce Nikki Farmston who runs a nonprofit organization based on peer support. We explore how program implementation rolls out, including the experience of hiring staff, providing trainings, designing logic models, and conducting evaluations. Use this chapter to explore the role of a manager in a health promotion program.
- In Chapter 8, we take you into the planning process for a townhall event. In addition to exploring compositions of planning committees, we review the importance of establishing mission statements, goals, and objectives. Use this chapter to explore the '*do's and don'ts*' of writing objectives.

- In Chapter 9, we introduce Rose Staybrite and showcase her journey in starting and supporting a Recovery Café. We explore fundraising and marketing concepts, as well as considerations for locating physical spaces for people to congregate.

- In Chapter 10, we introduce Jeannette O'Augusta and Craig Boullion who jump into community organizing and find success in the process. We introduce concepts like community readiness, gatekeeping, and cultural competency. Use this chapter to understand advocacy for public health issues.

- In Chapter 11, we take you through the process of establishing a Trauma-Informed Recovery-Oriented System of Care. We explore communication strategies used to motivate group participants, speak with the public, and convince stakeholders on the interconnectedness of trauma and substance use. Consider this chapter a deep dive into the root of addiction.

In addition to these 11 main chapters, we have a series of special-focus chapters, tailored to explore specific issues in program planning, including hiring external vendors and working with volunteers. Finally, we conclude with a special-focus chapter that discusses relevant concepts about treatment and recovery from substance use disorders.

DISCUSSION QUESTIONS

1. Try to draw a graphic representing the macro, mezzo, and micro levels of ecological systems in your own life. What does your graphic look like? How are the levels connected to each other?

2. We have highlighted the impact of substance misuse on families. What are other ways substance use affects our society?

3. Is the opioid crisis possible to solve? Can you imagine multifaceted solutions to address the opioid crisis that would be culturally appropriate, politically acceptable, technically feasible, and financially possible? Dream big!

REFERENCES

Ashrafioun, L., Dambra, C. M., & Blondell, R. D. (2011). Parental prescription opioid abuse and the impact on children. The American Journal of Drug and Alcohol Use, 37(6), 532–536. https://doi.org/10.3109/00952990.2011.600387

Barnard, M. & McKeganey, N. (2004). The impact of parental problem drug use on children: What is the problem and what can be done to help? Addiction, 99(5), 552–559. https://doi.org/10.1111/j.1360-0443.2003.00664.x

Barnes, G. M., Reifman, A. S., Farrell, M. P., & Dintcheff, B. A. (2000). The effects of parenting on the development of adolescent alcohol misuse: A six-wave latent growth model. Journal of Marriage and Family, 62(1), 175–186. https://doi.org/10.1111/j.17413737.2000.00175.x

Boyd, G. M., & Faden, V. (2002). Overview. Journal of Studies on Alcohol, 14, 6–13.

Bullinger, L. & Wing, C. (2019). How many children live with adults with opioid use disorder? Children and Youth Services Review, 104, 1. https://doi.org/10.1016/j.childyouth.2019.06.016

Callero, P. L. (2017). The Myth of Individualism: How Social Forces Shape Our Lives. Washington, DC: Rowman & Littlefield.

Centers for Disease Control (2021). *High School YRBS*. https://nccd.cdc.gov/youthonline/App

Centers for Disease Control (2022). *Death Rates Maps and Graphs*. https://www.cdc.gov/drugoverdose/deaths/index.html

Centers for Disease Control (2023). *Provisional Drug Overdose Death Counts*. https://www.cdc.gov/nchs/nvss/vsrr/drug-overdose-data.htm

Chassin, L., Sher, K., Hussong, A., & Curran, P. (2013). The developmental psychopathology of alcohol use and alcohol disorders: Research achievements and future directions. Development and Psychopathology, 25(4), 1567–1584. https://doi.org/10.1017/S0954579413000771

Comiskey, C. (2013). A 3 year national longitudinal study comparing drug treatment outcomes for opioid users with and without children in their custodial care at intake. Journal of Substance Abuse Treatment, 44(1), 90–96. https://doi.org/10.1016/j.jsat.2012.04.002

Cook, A., Spinazzola, J., Ford, J., Lanktree, C., Blaustein, M., Cloitre, M., . . . & Van der Kolk, B. (2017). Complex trauma in children and adolescents. Psychiatric Annals, 35(5), 390. https://doi.org/10.3928/00485713-20050501-05

Cox, R. W. (1981). Social forces, states and world orders: Beyond international relations theory. Millennium, 10(2), 126–155.

Edlunda, M. J., Forman-Hoffman, V. L., Winder, C. R., Heller, D. C., Kroutil, L. A., Lipari, R. N., & Colpec, L. J. (2015). Opioid abuse and depression in adolescents: Results from the national survey on drug use and health. Drug and Alcohol Dependence, 152, 131–138. https://doi.org/10.1016/j.drugalcdep.2015.04.010

Elkins, D. J. (1979). A cause in search of its effect, or what does political culture explain? Comparative Politics, 11(2), 127–145.

Estola, M. (2001). A dynamic theory of a firm: An application of 'economic forces'. Advances in Complex Systems, 4(01), 163–176.

Fischer, J. L., & Lyness, K. P. (2005). Families Coping with Alcohol and Substance Abuse. https://www.semanticscholar.org/paper/Families-Coping-With-Alcohol-and-Substance-Abuse-Fischer-Lyness/caf53d88048e4390d9c96728699e3e5b04e02d36.

Garrett, J. & Landau, J. (2007). Family motivation to change: a major factor in engaging alcoholics in treatment. Alcoholism Treatment Quarterly, 25(1-2), 65–83.

Godsall, R. E., Jurkovic, G. J., Emshoff, J., Anderson, L., & Stanwyck, D. (2004). Why some kids do well in bad situations: Relation of parental alcohol misuse and parentification to children's self-concept. Substance Use & Misuse, 39(5), 789–809. https://doi.org/10.1081/JA-120034016

Gonidec, P.F (1981). The Bases of Political Forces. Dordrecht: Springer. https://doi.org/10.1007/978-94-009-8902-3_2

Grella, C., Needell, B., Shi, Y., & Hser, Y. (2009). Do drug treatment services predict reunification outcomes of mothers and their children in child welfare? Journal of Substance Abuse Treatment, 36(3), 278–293. https://doi.org/10.1016/j.jsat.2008.06.010

Guo, J., Hawkins, J., Hill, K., & Abbott, R. (2001). Childhood and adolescent predictors of alcohol abuse and dependence in young adulthood. Journal of Studies on Alcohol, 62(6), 754–762. https://doi.org/10.15288/jsa.2001.62.754

Hedegaard, H., Minino, A., & Warner, M. (2020). Drug Overdose Deaths in the United States, 1999-2019. National Center for Health Statistics, 394. https://www.cdc.gov/nchs/products/databriefs/db394.htm

Hedegaard, H., Minino, A., Spencer, M., & Warner, M. (2021). Drug Overdose Deaths in the United States, 1999–2020. National Center for Health Statistics.

Heilbroner, R. L. & Thurow, L. (1998). Economics Explained: Everything You Need to Know About How the Economy Works and Where It's Going. Simon and Schuster.

Henderson, C. E., Rowe, C. L., Dakof, G. A., Hawes, S. W., & Liddle, H. A. (2009). Parenting practices as mediators of treatment effects in an early-intervention trial of multidimensional family therapy. The American Journal of Drug and Alcohol Abuse, 35(4), 220–226. https://doi.org/10.1080/00952990903005890

Hirai, A.H., Ko, J.Y, Owens, P.L., Stocks, C., & Patrick, S.W. (2021). Neonatal abstinence syndrome and maternal opioid related diagnoses in the US, 2010–2017. JAMA—Journal of the American Medical Association, 325(2), 146–155. https://doi.org/10.1001/jama.2020.24991

Hoagland, G.W. et al. (2019). Ending HIV in America: Policy and Program Insights from Local Health Agencies and Providers. Washington, DC.: Bipartisan Policy Center.

Khan, N., Bateman, B., Landon, J., & Gagne, J. (2019). Association of opioid overdose with opioid prescriptions to family members. JAMA Internal Medicine, 179(9), 1186–1192. https://doi.org/10.1001/jamainternmed.2019.1064

Leonard, K., & Eiden, R. (2007). Marital and family processes in the context of alcohol use and alcohol disorders. Annual Review of Clinical Psychology, 3(1), 285–310. https://doi.org/10.1146/annurev.clinpsy.3.022806.091424

Lewis, V., & Allen-Byrd, L. (2007). Coping strategies for the stagesof family recovery. In J. L. Fischer, M. Mulsow, & A. W. Korinek (Eds.), Familial Responses to Alcohol Problems (pp. 105–124). Binghamton, NY: Hawthorn Press.

Leza, L., Siria, S., Lopez-Goni, J., Fernandez-Montalvo, J. (2021). Adverse childhood experiences (ACEs) and substance use disorder (SUD): A scoping review. Drug and Alcohol Dependence, 221(1). https://www.sciencedirect.com/science/article/abs/pii/S0376871621000582

Luo, F., Li, M., & Florence, C. (2021). State-level economic costs of opioid use disorder and opioid overdose – United States, 2017. Morbidity and Mortality Weekly Report, 70(15), 541–546. https://www.cdc.gov/mmwr/volumes/70/wr/mm7015a1.htm#:~:text=The%20economic%20cost%20of%20the,at%20%24550%20billion%20(3).

Martins, S., Keyes, K., Storr, C., Zhu, H., & Chilcoat, H. (2009). Pathways between nonmedical opioid use/dependence and psychiatric disorders: Results from the national epidemiologic survey on alcohol and related conditions. Drug and Alcohol Dependence, 103(1–2), 16–24.

Maté, G. (2010). In the Realm of the Hungry Ghosts: Close Encounters with Addiction. Berkeley, CA: North Atlantic Books.

Messler, E. C., Quevillon, R. P., & Simons, J. S. (2014). The effect of perceived parental approval of drinking on alcohol use and problems. Journal of Alcohol and Drug Education, 58(1), 44.

Mirick, R. G. & Steenrod, S. A. (2016). Opioid use disorder, attachment, and parenting: Key concerns for practitioners. Child and Adolescent Social Work Journal, 33(6), 547–557. https://doi.org/10.1007/s10560-016-0449-1

Mitsi, V. & Zachariou, V. (2016). Modulation of pain, nociception, and analgesia by the brain reward center. Neuroscience, 338, 81–92. https://doi.org/10.1016/j.neuroscience.2016.05.017

Monnat, S. M. & Rigg, K. K. (2016). Examining rural/urban differences in prescription opioid misuse among US adolescents. Journal of Rural Health, 32(2), 204–18. https://doi.org/10.1111/jrh.12141

Murphy, S. (2021). The cost of opioid use disorder and the value of aversion. Drug and Alcohol Dependency, 217. https://www.ncbi.nlm.nih.gov/pmc/articles/PMC7737485/#:~:text=and%20stakeholder%20perspective.-,The%20mean%20present%20value%20of%20averting%20an%20OUD%2C%20across%20all,from%20a%20healthcare%20sector%20perspective.

National Center for Drug Abuse Statistics (2023). Drug Overdose Death Rates. https://drugabusestatistics.org/drug-overdose-deaths/#:~:text=Opioid%20Overdose%20Death%20Rates,than%20136%20Americans%20every%20day.

National Center for Health Statistics (2021). Wide-ranging Online Data for Epidemiologic Research (WONDER). Atlanta, GA: CDC. http://wonder.cdc.gov.

O'Farrell, T. & Clements, K. (2012). Review of outcome research on marital and family therapy in treatment for alcoholism. Journal of Marital Family Therapy, 38(1), 122–144.

Peisch, V., Sullivan, A. D., Breslend, N. L., Benoit, R., Sigmon, S. C., Forehand, G. L., . . . & Forehand, R. (2018). Parental opioid abuse: A review of child outcomes, parenting, and parenting interventions. Journal of Child and Family Studies, 27(7), 2082–2099. https://doi.org/10.1007/s10826-018-1061-0

Rogers, C.J., Pakdaman, S., Forster, M., Sussman, S., Grigsby, T.J., Victoria, J., & Unger, J.B. (2022). Effects of multiple adverse childhood experiences on substance use in young adults: A review of the literature. Drug and Alcohol Dependence, 234, 1. https://www.sciencedirect.com/science/article/abs/pii/S0376871622001442

Schempf, A. H., & Strobino, D. M. (2009). Drug use and limited prenatal care: An examination of responsible barriers. American Journal of Obstetrics and Gynecology, 200(4), 1–10. https://doi.org/10.1016/j.ajog.2008.10.055

Schiff, D., & Patrick, S. (2017). Treatment of opioid use disorder during pregnancy and cases of neonatal abstinence syndrome. JAMA Pediatrics, 171(7), 707–707. https://doi.org/10.1001/jamapediatrics.2017.0854

Scholl, L., Seth, P., Kariisa, M., Wilson, N., & Baldwin, G. (2019). Drug and opioid-involved overdose deaths—United States, 2013–2017. Morbidity and Mortality Weekly Report, 67(51–52), 1419.

Scott, C.K., Dennis, M.L., Grella, C.E. et al. The impact of the opioid crisis on U.S. state prison systems. Health Justice 9, 17 (2021). https://doi.org/10.1186/s40352-021-00143-9

Substance Abuse and Mental Health Services Administration (2022). Key substance use and mental health indicators in the United States: Results from the 2021 National Survey on Drug Use and Health (HHS Publication No. PEP22-07-01-005, NSDUH Series H-57). Center for Behavioral Health Statistics and Quality, Substance Abuse and Mental Health Services Administration. https://www.samhsa.gov/data/report/2021-nsduh-annualnational-report.

Suchman, N., Pajulo, M., DeCoste, C., & Mayes, L. (2006). Parenting interventions for drug-dependent mothers and their young children: The case for an attachment-based approach. Family Relations, 55(2), 211–226. https://doi.org/10.1111/j.1741-3729.2006.00371.x doi:10.1016/j.drugalcdep.2009.01.019

Spehr, M., Coddington, J., Ahmed, A., & Jones, E. (2017). Parental opioid abuse: barriers to care, policy, and implications for primary care pediatric providers. Journal of Pediatric Health Care, 31(6), 695–702.

Swadi, H. (1999). Individual risk factors for adolescent substance use. Drug and Alcohol Dependence, 55(3), 209–224.

Taplin, S., & Mattick, R. P. (2015). The nature and extent of child protection involvement among heroin-using mothers in treatment: High rates of reports, removals at birth and children in care. Drug and Alcohol Review, 34(1), 31–37. https://doi.org/10.1111/dar.12165

US Department of Justice—Drug Enforcement Administration & US Department of Education—Office of Safe & Healthy Students (2017). Growing Up Drug Free: A Parent's Guide to Prevention. https://www.dea.gov/sites/default/files/2018-06/growing-up-drug-free-2017.pdf

Wexelblatt, S., McAllister, J., Nathan, A., & Hall, E. (2018). Opioid neonatal abstinence syndrome: An overview. Clinical Pharmacology & Therapeutics, 103(6), 979–981. https://doi.org/10.1002/cpt.958

Young, J. L. & Martin, P. R. (2012) Treatment of opioid dependence in the setting of pregnancy. Psychiatric Clinics of North America, 35(2), 441–460. https://doi.org/10.1016/j.psc.2012.03.008

CHAPTER

1

COMMUNITY HEALTH NEEDS ASSESSMENT

COLLECTING DATA TO INFORM INTERVENTIONS

In this chapter, we highlight how a formalized needs assessment provides a systematic way to gather and analyze data to begin to solve community problems. Program planning is more effective when the needs and voices of community members, and not merely the goals of administrators and practitioners, are incorporated into the process.

Flynn Mosi, Director of Community Outreach for a large nonprofit area hospital, was sitting comfortably in a polo shirt, smiling generously across the table. He was talking about the hospital's ongoing community health needs assessment. Flynn loved that conducting a needs assessment was part of his job. Specifically, he explained, he loved being part of connecting the hospital to his home town in a way that improved the overall health of the community. Additionally, his efforts ensured that the hospital would maintain its tax-exempt status, as each nonprofit area hospital was required to conduct an assessment every three years.

Health Promotion Planning: Learning from the Accounts of Public Health Practitioners,
First Edition. Jean Marie S. Place, Jonel Thaller, and Scott S. Hall.
© 2024 John Wiley & Sons, Inc. Published 2024 by John Wiley & Sons, Inc.

Flynn explained that the purpose of a **community health needs assessment** was to identify community health needs and inform the planning and development of an implementation strategy to address these needs. In his county, community health needs could include high rates of diabetes, accidents, or behavioral health issues, among many other health problems. They could also include barriers to care, such as lack of accessibility, availability, or affordability of services. The *Patient Protection and Affordable Care Act*, or "Obamacare," was behind the push to assess and plan for community health needs in Flynn's region. It required that Flynn and his team collect a wide range of data, compare the relative importance of multiple health problems, and set priorities to address the top needs in the community. Flynn flashed a smile and excitedly shared that the needs assessment process would take place in three phases: (1) data collection, (2) data analysis, and (3) intervention planning.

FOCUS GROUPS AS A MEANS OF DATA COLLECTION

Flynn and his team began the needs assessment process by conducting focus groups to learn about the community's health needs. They were in the process of conducting three focus groups at different times and on different days of the week within a two-month period. The people first invited to participate were change agents in the community, rich with connections to the wider population. Attendees included directors of nonprofits, public health practitioners, neighborhood association leaders, healthcare providers, outreach specialists, business owners, and case workers.

Focus groups, or group interviews, are a research method used to elicit people's opinions, feelings, beliefs, insights, attitudes, and perspectives on a selected topic. Focus groups are qualitative in nature, meaning a facilitator uses a guide to ask open-ended questions to a small group (usually between 7 and 10 people) to learn what group members think about the topic. In a needs assessment, focus groups can be used to identify a variety of needs in a community.

Some focus groups use *purposive sampling*, which involves recruiting people who meet certain criteria, such as those who share a similar life experience or demographic background. Results from focus group discussions with specific populations can be compared to find similarities and differences among groups.

A skilled moderator who can create a comfortable atmosphere and elicit responses to questions is necessary for conducting a focus group. A co-moderator can also help by drawing attention to group dynamics that the lead moderator might overlook. With participants' consent, focus groups should be audio-recorded so that data can be transcribed to written text to facilitate analysis.

Remember that results emerging from focus groups might not be generalizable to other groups because of purposive sampling where participants are selected based on certain characteristics or criteria.

Flynn described a practical matter in forming the focus groups, that of making sure the groups were neither too big nor too small. He had learned to keep each group between 12 and 15 people. He explained why: "In a focus group of 30 people, 20 of the people never get to talk, so you're not hearing from a large portion of people. But, if groups are too small, one person feels like they can take center stage. They'll begin to drive the whole meeting and dominate the discussion. That's not good either." He continued, "For these reasons, I've found that 12–15 people is a pretty good size, and everybody gets a chance to talk." Flynn planned to use purposive sampling to recruit professionals to attend the first focus group. Later in the month, he would invite members of the lay public to attend a second focus group.

On a hot day in April, Flynn spoke with 15 attendees over video conference to learn more about what they see as the most pressing health issues in the community. The goal of the group was to consider multiple health challenges, and debate and reflect on which ones were most important, which ones were changeable, and which should be the focus of community change efforts. From this effort, he anticipated a short list of more urgent issues would emerge and become visible from the dozens of health problems that existed in the community.

To get the meeting started, Flynn encouraged everyone to briefly introduce themselves. Then, he promptly outlined how the focus group would proceed. First, he would share recent health statistics – secondary data from federal-, state-, and county-level surveys – to paint a picture of the community's health needs. Then he would ask for feedback and reflections on the data shared.

Secondary data is data already collected by someone else for a different purpose and made available for the public to access through online datasets. It includes existing data generated from large government institutions, healthcare facilities, or other data collection organizations, and available in books, on websites, or in journal articles or other publications.

Primary data is information collected firsthand, generally via survey, questionnaire, qualitative interview, or focus group.

The secondary data presented to focus group participants in the video conference included demographics of the county (e.g. age ranges, education levels, ethnicity), health status among residents, and factors that influence health status. The data were pulled from the Robert Wood Johnson County Health Rankings, the state Department of Health, US census track data, as well as other state, federal, and foundation sources. Data on the county included the following:

- The percent of residents with a disability was higher than state and national averages.
- Poverty rates for residents were above the state and national averages. Poverty rates for Black and Hispanic (or Latino) residents were generally above the poverty rate of White residents.
- Unemployment rates were above state and national averages.
- The percentage of people uninsured was above the national average.
- Crime rates were below state averages.
- Rates of mortality for diabetes in the county were significantly higher than state averages.
- The county had overall cancer mortality and lung cancer mortality rates that exceeded state averages.
- Rates of women who smoked during pregnancy were more than 50% higher than the state average.
- Several census tracts in the county were designated as food deserts.
- The percent of children in poverty in the county was 22.2%.

Flynn explained why he started the focus group by presenting secondary data. "I had to encourage participants to talk about what data points stood out as well as what was notably absent in the reporting." Secondary data can only say so much, and Flynn intended that the focus group discussion would fill in any **data gaps** to better understand the needs of the population. Thus, while secondary data was used to launch the focus group, the discussion would become a new source of primary data about the health of the community, with participants providing feedback on whether the statistics shared reflected the true needs of their community. What things stood out in the statistical picture? What was not presented that should have been?

As the focus group proceeded, Flynn asked open-ended questions to deepen the conversation and prompt the attendees to further consider community needs. He asked the following questions: What needs are you personally seeing? What do people in our community struggle with? What do we need to focus on to help people in our community? These questions were variations of the core question of a needs assessment: What are the needs of the target population? In this case, the target population was referring to residents of the county.

Within the focus group, one attendee suggested lack of access to healthy foods was a problem, and another noted community issues with financial literacy. Others rallied around mental health issues and shared stories to emphasize their point. "Lack of birth control," another small cohort insisted. Addiction and substance misuse was mentioned again and again, including addiction to prescription pain killers, and everyone agreed COVID-19 exacerbated health disparities.

Comments varied and people spoke adamantly while Flynn maintained an objective ear and calmly added responses to a list. The secondary data that initially kicked-off the focus group discussion was quantitative in nature, represented as statistics, ratios, and numbers, but the discussion that followed was qualitative in nature, lending deeper insight to the statistical picture by including attendees' multi-faceted perspectives, thoughts, reflections, and opinions.

Quantitative data is numerical and can be measured, counted, and quantified. Quantitative methods can include physiological biomarkers, such as blood pressure or body mass index, as well as social surveys and questionnaires.

Qualitative data is not numerical in nature and is often expressed as words instead of numbers. Qualitative methods include single subject interviews, focus group discussions, and scientific observation. Qualitative data is often used to describe people's thoughts, experiences, and behaviors.

Flynn posed other questions, pulling in additional features of a needs assessment: Why do these needs exist? What factors determine or create these needs? Which subgroups within the target population have the greatest need? More conversation ensued and people spoke animatedly, making the case that generational poverty and low socioeconomic status were at the root of health issues (i.e. how can people find time to eat healthy food if they are working three jobs? one attendee insisted) and others added that a lack of education, knowledge, and awareness perpetuates health problems. Some people emphasized "pill mills" as a root of the opioid crisis, where facilities prescribe or dispense of narcotics inappropriately for nonmedical reasons.

While the focus group discussion mainly centered on identifying the health needs of the community, Flynn emphasied how it was also important to consider the community's capacity to address the expressed needs. What community resources were available to address the needs? One focus group participant thought food security was a critical need, and to consider meeting this need, the group discussed community resources that existed to address food insecurity, such as a mobile grocery truck that rotated weekly to low-income neighborhoods or the cell phone app that helped residents navigate to free food resources in the area. Flynn encouraged more discussion by asking: "What is currently being done to resolve identified needs in our community? How well have needs been addressed in the past?" Flynn expressed that knowing what resources exist among individuals, organizations, and communities - and what is lacking - can point to areas for improvement.

Finally, Flynn paused the conversation, directed participants to the chat box available via the video conference platform, and pasted the group's list of expressed community needs into the box. "Scroll through the list," he said, "and see if your top perceived need changed based on the conversation." He continued, "Then, you should select the top three needs from your perspective, verbally state these needs, and add nothing more." Just like that, the lively discussion ended – the preferences would be tallied, calculated, and stored away until the final report, combined with other sources of primary and secondary data, would be released publicly. The result would provide the top needs of the population, as determined by a variety of stakeholders and sources.

One common framework for community health needs assessment is called the *Mobilizing for Action through Planning and Partnerships* (MAPP). MAPP introduces four specific areas of assessment for public health practitioners to consider when assessing community needs:

- The *Community Themes and Strengths Assessment* asks questions such as "What is important to the community?" "How is quality of life perceived in our community?" and "What assets do we have that can be used to improve community health?"

- The *Local Public Health System Assessment* focuses on questions such as "What are the components, activities, competencies, and capacities of our local public health system?" and "How are essential services being provided to our community?"

- The *Community Health Status Assessment* looks at questions such as "How healthy are our residents?" and "What does the health status of our community look like?"

- The *Forces of Change Assessment* seeks to identify impending, external changes that affect the context of the public health system. Questions include, "What is occurring or might occur in legislation, technology, or other areas that could affect the health of our community and the local public health system?" and "What specific threats or opportunities are generated by these occurrences?"

Guidance and toolkits for each of the assessments are available from the National Association of County and City Health Officials at https://www.naccho. org/programs/public-health-infrastructure/performance-improvement/ community-health-assessment/mapp/phase-3-the-four-assessments.

SURVEYS AS A MEANS OF DATA COLLECTION

Apart from the focus groups, a quantitative survey was also administered to individuals across the community to supplement the information from the focus groups. The same survey was distributed across the state so that data collected in one area could be comparable to data from another, providing insight into where counties ranked on different health indicators. Individuals who received the survey request were asked to quantitatively rank different health problems from most important to least important.

Questions on needs assessment surveys generally include different categories of data, such as the following (NACCHO, 2023a):

- Demographic characteristics, like age, gender, race, and ethnicity
- Socioeconomic characteristics, like income, education, and employment
- Health resource availability, like number of licensed and credentialed providers, as well as measures of access, utilization, cost, and quality of health care services
- Quality of life, measured by reports of life, community, and healthcare satisfaction
- Behavioral risk factors, like substance use, nutrition and exercise, safety, and screenings
- Environmental health indicators, like clean air and water, safely prepared foods, exposure to hazardous substances, and unintentional injuries
- Social and mental health status, including violence in the home or community

- Maternal and child health status, like birth outcomes and mortality for infants and children, adolescent pregnancy, and maternal access and utilization of care
- Death, illness, and injury status, like mortality and morbidity rates
- Infectious disease, including diseases transmitted through person-to-person contact or through shared use of contaminated instruments
- Sentinel events, like vaccine-preventable illness, late-stage cancer diagnosis, and other unexpected syndromes or infections

Flynn talked about the decision behind mailing paper surveys to participants versus sending a digital version through email. At first, they tried both methods, but the results were skewed toward younger people when they used email. "It felt a little biased," Flynn explained. After all, he could only send the survey through email to contacts whom he already knew. It was important to have a sample beyond fellow colleagues or friends. They tried distributing the survey link as a pop-up ad on the local newspaper website where viewers could click to take the survey. Still, he said, "that's biased towards people who are looking at that website. You're missing a lot of people."

Posting the link on a website for internal hospital employees was similarly biased. While the strategy generated many responses among employees, Flynn emphasized, "I didn't have that same access with the factory down the street," meaning that factory workers were unintentionally excluded from the sample because he did not have an easy way to get the survey in front of them. Flynn recognized that ideally participants included in a sample are reflective of the general population in knowledge, attitudes, and behaviors, but the methods Flynn tried generated a **nonprobability sample,** meaning the participants were not representative of the larger population. Flynn was accessing a **nonprobability convenience sample** as he selected potential participants that were easiest to reach, based on who he had access to, and this sample was unfortunately not representative of actual community demographics.

Even though the team eventually transitioned to paper surveys, they still struggled to obtain a **representative sample**, or a group of people with backgrounds varied enough to be reflective of the larger community. Flynn recalled, "I literally went out to canvas neighborhoods with the paper survey. I went to community meetings and passed out the survey, but, again, that was biased towards who I knew and who I had a working relationship with." Finally, they bought a cross-sectional list of contact information for households across the city and mailed the survey to those addresses, with a request that people complete the survey and mail it back. However, even this attempt to eliminate bias only resulted in roughly 11% of households responding. By using the list of city households, Flynn was attempting to use a **probability sample**, where he systematically and randomly selected households as potential participants. This method gave each person on the list an equal chance of being selected. Regrettably, not very many people who were asked to complete the survey actually did.

MOVING FROM DATA COLLECTION TO ANALYSIS AND ACTION

Information shared by participants in the focus group and collected from surveys was paired with in-depth interviews from the county health director, CEOs of local health centers, and other nonprofit leaders. These sources formed the primary data. Secondary data were used to help identify the areas and sub-populations most in need of intervention.

Flynn noted the importance of sub-analyses to assess differences among different groups in a population. "There is some secondary data specific to sub-populations, whether it's the elderly, or race-based, or gender-based, or based on zip codes." Those sub-analyses were important because "if we're going to do a program in the community, we're not going to do it where the obesity rate is 12%. We're going to look for where the obesity rate is 49.5%!" In other words, he strongly felt that programs should be designed for segments of the population most in need.

Some of the primary and secondary data in the final report included the following findings:

- Stakeholders identified mental health, poverty, health resources, and substance abuse as some of the most significant needs for residents of the community. In light of the COVID-19 pandemic, stakeholders also focused on isolation and its impact on mental health, lack of preventative health care, and racial and ethnic disparities as additional problems.
- The county was in the bottom quartile of state's counties for poor mental health days.
- It ranked in the bottom half of the state's counties for physical health and social determinants of health, including social and economic factors, unemployment, and children in poverty. It also had high vulnerability to transportation problems among residents.
- Additionally, the county was among the very worst in the state for quality of life, mental and physical health days, child poverty, income inequality, and severe housing problems.

Rather than being dismayed, Flynn felt energized by these facts. He asked, "What are we going to do to address the needs that we find? That's the beauty of the whole thing. It spurs hospitals into action."

After completing the data collection process, an external vendor was hired to sift through the data and conduct a thorough analysis, boiling down the data points and providing a list of the needs that arose at least two or more times through different data collection methods.

The top seven needs were as follows:

1. Access to Healthcare Services
2. Drug and Substance Abuse (including Opioids and Alcohol)
3. Food Insecurity and Healthy Eating
4. Mental Health
5. Obesity, Diabetes, and Physical Inactivity
6. Smoking and Tobacco Usage
7. Social Determinants of Health

The hospital administrative boards approved the report, and Flynn began designing a plan to address the most pressing needs. He explained, "We don't have to address every need. We don't have to address them all by ourselves. The key is that we do address the ones that we think are the most pressing." He understood that focusing on top needs, as opposed to *every* need, builds support for utilizing resources in areas where the most impact is likely to happen (McKenzie et al., 2017). Flynn described meeting with his direct supervisor, the chief of staff, and the presidents of other in-network hospitals to review the data and determine which needs could be most effectively addressed. Addressing poverty, for example, was mentioned multiple times as a community need, but it was not chosen as a need that the hospital network felt it could successfully impact.

During the planning process, when setting priorities, it is important to consider whether resources are available to address the expressed needs. Program planners must consider how much control they have over the issue and whether they have sufficient knowledge of the issue. Thus, in a context of limited resources, stakeholders may need to coalesce support around specific needs that have been prioritized, especially if there are not sufficient resources to address all needs.

According to the National Association of County and City Health Officials (NACCHO, 2023b), the following criteria are helpful for prioritizing health issues:

- *Size* – How many people are affected?

- *Seriousness* – How many deaths, disabilities, or hospitalizations are a result of the problem?
- *Trends* – Is it getting worse or better?
- *Equity* – Are some groups affected more?
- *Intervention* – Is there a proven strategy?
- *Values* – Does the community care about it?
- *Social determinants* – Are there social and economic conditions that are at the root of the issue?

The resources to address poverty were beyond what the hospital could commit to. But the hospital did have resources and strategies to address other needs. Flynn noted that there was no need to reinvent the wheel when it came to designing strategies: "If we have an existing program that's already in place, and we're getting measurement from that, then let's put that down as a strategy." Flynn further described the importance of not duplicating effort as he related the following story:

> I drove conversations with different departments. I basically would say, "Hey, here's what we learned as a community health need, what's going on with behavioral health in your world, and what can you translate into some strategy?" In that process of that detective work, I find out that we're about to roll out a program at our emergency department where we have folks that are basically what are called peer recovery coaches, and so, boom, that becomes a strategy!

Flynn was exploring intervention strategies when he visited with different departments, inquiring about the programs that existed within each unit. Flynn was looking at what health promotion programs were presently available to the target population and if the programs were being utilized (McKenzie et al., 2017). These fact-finding questions were crucial before designing new interventions.

Through Flynn's networking, he learned that location was one reason why some programs were not well-utilized. For some individuals on the southside of the city, for example, navigating the bus line to arrive at a northside location was too difficult. The times that programs were offered mattered, too, especially for people who worked variable shifts or were not able to access a program during working hours. Other programs had qualifying criteria for enrollment, such as insurance or age requirements. Cost was a barrier for many low-income individuals who simply could not afford interventions that had a price tag.

As ambitious as ever, Flynn did indeed pick all seven needs and planned how to intervene in each of them. He stated, "I immediately went to work on those strategies for implementation," but he acknowledged, "We're not able to solve these issues, but we can create strategies that at least address them and make a dent. We're trying to find where we can measure the impact along the way."

Because substance misuse was identified as a top need from the community health needs assessment, Flynn and his team planned and developed intervention strategies that included enhanced SBIRT screening. SBIRT is a screening tool and refers to *screening, brief intervention and referral to treatment*. It is an approach that healthcare providers can implement in their practices to identify and help patients with problematic substance use or those at risk for developing a substance use disorder. Flynn wanted to see this screening tool deployed among every patient seen at the Family Medicine Residency clinic.

Another intervention strategy Flynn intended to develop, based on the results of the needs assessment, was to screen and refer patients at the hospital's pain management program for behavioral health counseling. Beyond the clinical setting, Flynn was planning intervention strategies for the community at large by aiming to bring a parenting and family support program to the county. Other intervention strategies included evening stress management groups, middle-school prevention initiatives, and large-scale awareness campaigns for mental health.

Flynn and his team would have two years to carry out the action plan before the community health needs assessment process started over. In two years, he would be back at the drawing board collecting another round of primary data to be used for planning future interventions.

DISCUSSION QUESTIONS

1. Do you think planning is something with a single beginning and ending? Explain.

2. How might data from a focus group differ from data gathered in a one-on-one interview?

3. What are the advantages and disadvantages of focus group discussions versus one-on-one interviewing?

4. What are the advantages and disadvantages of collecting and using qualitative versus quantitative data?

5. What biases might emerge to impact data when conducting interviews or administering surveys to community members?

6. How would you ensure that all voices in a community are heard in an assessment? Is that even possible, or desirable?

7. What are some advantages and disadvantages of setting priorities based on how commonly certain topics are mentioned by a group?

8. What value can come from comparing data from one county to another? In what ways might this data be unhelpful or misleading?

9. Which would be more valuable – making a "dent" in eight different problems or coming close to solving one or two problems? How would you decide?

ACTIVITIES

1. Consider the primary data (local focus groups and survey results) as well as the secondary data (county, state, and federal statistics) included in this community health needs assessment. Consider how well the two types of data do or do not match up. What opportunities or insights might be overlooked by those designing interventions if either the primary or secondary data are unavailable?

2. Do a web search to find a list of community problems in your state or county. Investigate how this list was put together. What steps were taken to gather and use data, and how did that compare to what you read in this chapter? If the list is rank ordered, see if you can identify a logic or reasoning behind the ordering. If not ranked, how might you go about ranking them?

REFERENCES

McKenzie, J., Neiger, B., & Thackeray, R. (2017). *Planning, Implementing, and Evaluating Health Promotion Programs: A Primer*. USA: Pearson.

National Association of City and County Health Organizations. (2023a). *Phase 3: Collecting and Analyzing Data*. https://www.naccho.org/programs/public-health-infrastructure/performance-improvement/community-health-assessment/mapp/phase-3-the-four-assessments

National Association of City and County Health Organizations. (2023b). *Phase 4: Identifying and Prioritizing Strategic Issues*. https://www.naccho.org/programs/public-health-infrastructure/performance-improvement/community-health-assessment/mapp/phase-4-identify-strategic-issues

CHAPTER

FATALITY REVIEW BOARD

IDENTIFYING RISK FACTORS FOR POOR HEALTH OUTCOMES

In this chapter, we illustrate the importance of understanding risk factors associated with health outcomes. Data collected and combined from multiple perspectives facilitates well-rounded program planning and can inform future prevention programs.

Kim, age 26, unemployed, died of a heroin overdose a few months after her fiancé died the same way. They were using the substance in a tent that served as their home.

Steve, age 42, father of four, after a stint in prison, overdosed on opioids and cocaine. He said his wife had cheated on him and drove him to drugs.

Lafina, age 55, was found in a hotel room, blood alcohol level off the charts, used needle found in the trash, missing her wallet and cell phone. There was suspicion that her death was orchestrated as retribution for a gang shooting incident. Her criminal history filled multiple

Health Promotion Planning: Learning from the Accounts of Public Health Practitioners,
First Edition. Jean Marie S. Place, Jonel Thaller, and Scott S. Hall.

pages of the community corrections report. Her oldest son was serving time for his own noteworthy record.

These three deaths, among many others, would be discussed in detail by a local fatality review team, convened by the county to identify and understand how various risk factors may have contributed to these untimely deaths and note where there were missed opportunities for intervention. The findings would be used to develop and enhance prevention and intervention programming.

Fatality review teams began to form across the Unites States throughout the 1980s to review the causes of child deaths. They were known as Child Death Reviews (CDRs). By 2001, all states had some form of a CDR.

In 2002, the US Department of Health and Human Services funded what would become the National Center for Fatality Review and Prevention (NCFRP). As a result, a wide variety of fatality review teams have emerged, focusing on specific types of victims, such as maternal fatalities, teen fatalities, intimate partner homicide fatalities, and fetal infant fatalities. More recently, fatality review procedures have been applied to investigating suicide and overdose fatalities to help generate prevention strategies.

Teams vary in their approaches to sharing, analyzing, and drawing conclusions from data, and also operate at different levels (e.g. county, statewide, or private agency) depending on the state.

USING FATALITY REVIEW BOARDS TO ASSESS NEEDS

Fabiola Martin from the state Department of Health made an announcement to the group of interprofessional practitioners gathered in the room: "You'll need to decide whether you want to review suicide fatalities, or just overdose fatalities."

She paused to sense the collective inclination of the nine other people in the room, ranging from individuals from the local police department, county probation office, community corrections, addiction treatment clinic, local pharmacy, Department of Child Services, and other community institutions.

This was the inaugural meeting for the county's overdose and suicide fatality review team. The team would be systematically reviewing each drug-related death in the county – a population of roughly 115,000 – that had occurred in the past 12 months. The goal was to better understand the various risk factors that led to each death.

Risk factors are characteristics or influences that increase the chance of developing a disease (morbidity) or dying (mortality). Risk factors contribute to our understanding of a person's vulnerability to poor outcomes.

Protective factors are characteristics or influences that can lower the chance of developing poor health outcomes. Some protective factors can even reduce a risk factor's negative impact. They can be seen as positive countering effects that create resilience.

According to the Substance Abuse and Mental Health Services Administration (SAMHSA), effective substance use prevention focuses on reducing risk factors and strengthening protective factors.

Consider, for example, the three deceased individuals named above. The team would be attempting to learn what made them more likely to die of substance misuse than their neighbors or any other people with whom they had lived and worked. The team would begin by noting certain well-known **behavioral risk factors** that placed them at a higher likelihood for experiencing poor health outcomes, including intravenous (injection) drug use, criminal activity, smoking, certain family and relationship patterns, and the experience of grief. Other factors were also at play.

Environmental risk factors also contributed to their deaths. In these cases, environmental risk factors do not merely include factors related to the natural environment, such as polluted air or unclean water, but also include forces in the social and cultural environment that surround and affect communities, such as poverty and unemployment. Were these people affected by poverty? Did they have access to jobs that paid a living wage? These questions are focused on the *economic environment*.

Similarly, did they have access to affordable and nondiscriminatory health care services? Did they have transportation to arrive at these services? These questions refer to the *service environment*.

What about their interpersonal connection with prosocial peers and people who loved and supported them? Did they experience alienation through negative peer pressure or childhood trauma? These questions refer to the *social environment*.

Understanding the *political environment* is likewise important. Was their substance misuse seen as a criminal justice problem deserving of incarceration, or a public health issue that warranted medical and mental health treatment? In short, was their behavior criminalized or treated like the symptom of an illness?

Risk and protective factors do not exist in isolation. They interact and influence each other in relationships, in community settings, and in society at large. They also tend to be cumulative. For example, people with some risk factors have a greater chance of experiencing even more risk factors and are less likely to have protective factors. Early intervention reduces the impact of risk factors.

Risk and protective factors can also have an influence throughout a person's lifespan. **Adverse childhood experiences**, or **ACEs**, such as childhood abuse and neglect, can have an effect many years later, adding to a person's risk for chronic health problems, mental illness, and substance use in adulthood.

Gathering detailed information about avoidable deaths was necessary for the fatality review team to evaluate which types of risk factors contributed to each tragedy. The team's initial task was to assemble and examine a patchwork of data from their respective records, such as

1. death certificates
2. medical charts
3. police reports
4. autopsy/toxicology reports
5. obituaries
6. social service case files
7. Department of Child Services records

These various pieces of **data** would help the team detect common risk factors that may have played a role in each person's death. Fabiola recognized that data were at the heart of the process. She explained, "We need to have access to as many pieces of information as possible about the person who died so that we can get a more complete picture about what is going on, what went wrong. It's like putting together a puzzle."

Each team member represented a particular service sector from the community and painted the deceased individuals in a particular light. Within police reports, for example, a person was defined by their criminal behavior – an individual who had made a series of bad choices, all of them self-destructive and some of them significantly harmful to others. But obituaries told a different story – a person who was missed by their loved ones, who had memorable personality traits and hobbies. These life summaries provided the team with the names of relatives and loved ones whose records they could also access for the purpose of filling in missing information.

But Fabiola's question still hung in the air, unanswered. Did the team want to review suicide fatalities as well as overdose fatalities? What would be the purpose and scope of the review?

The team's collective decision about whether they should review either suicide fatalities or overdose fatalities was the first step in conducting their interprofessional analysis. The answer to this question was important, because where the team chose to fix their attention would influence the rest of their process. The occupants in the room remained mostly silent as they considered the question.

Fabiola emphasized, "We need to consider the implications of our decision because it'll impact how we sift through these records. How we focus our attention matters."

States or counties often vary in how they organize their fatality reviews. While most seem to review all cases that fall within their designated category (e.g. overdose or suicide fatality), some select specific themes for any given year. In the span of one year, teams may choose to only review the veterans who died from an overdose. But, during another year, they may only review individuals who had been recently released from jail. Such a shift in focus leads to recommendations related to very specific populations.

A few of the team members were professionally or personally acquainted with one another. However, this first meeting had begun without any form of introductions, rapport, or team building. A few individuals new to this professional network seemed reserved and reticent to speak without an understanding of the context of the meeting and the many perspectives and expert opinions contained within the room. Fabiola later reflected, "Usually it can be a bit uncomfortable at first as people adjust to what we are there to do."

A man from the Department of Community Corrections with a friendly demeanor was the first to speak up. Other members of the group, some of them key decision-makers in the community, followed suit, sharing their thoughts and ideas about how to proceed. A consensus emerged to consider both overdose and suicide fatalities since they are often interconnected and difficult to place in solely one category or another.

Once this was determined, Fabiola began an overview of the fatality review process. She explained that some states already had fatality review teams that focused on specific types of victims: domestic violence fatalities, maternal fatalities, teen fatalities, child fatalities, and fetal/infant fatalities. But applying this type of review to overdose and suicide fatalities, she noted, was just catching on. In 2018, their state became one of a handful nationally who had formed overdose fatality review teams. The federal Centers for Disease Control and Prevention distributed money to the state, and the county's local coordinating council for substance use prevention (CCSUP) had sought funds from the state Department of Health to support forming and sustaining a fatality review team. The team would meet monthly at the CCSUP offices. Not all counties received funding to review fatality cases – in some states there was only a single overdose fatality review team. A ripple of interest moved across the room – they were fortunate to be sitting in this room.

> Much of the funding for substance misuse prevention and intervention at the county level can be traced back to the state and then federal level. Given that states have a better grasp on localized service needs than the country, many national funding sources distribute funds at the state level and allow the states to distribute funding to counties as necessary.

SELF-CARE IS NEEDED IN PUBLIC HEALTH WORK

The mood of the room eventually fell into a solemn silence – people looked up from their phones, the rustling of papers ceased – when Fabiola lowered her voice, stating, "This is hard, emotionally draining work." The task, she explained, was not about judgment, but about trying to understand the person: the human being behind each mortality statistic was a person who was someone's child, grandchild, sibling, parent, or best friend. "It is important," she continued, "for people who work in emotionally challenging situations to monitor and nurture their own physical and mental health so they can continue to be available to serve others."

As if to reinforce the sober mood in the room, a police officer noted that in the past four weeks alone the county had seen three overdose fatalities and at least two drug-related suicides. Perhaps to lighten the mood, a woman pointed out that on the plus side they would be getting a free lunch, leading someone to wonder out loud, "Will I be more prone to getting sick to my stomach if I eat *before* or *after* reviewing the gut-wrenching details of each case?" People in the room welcomed the chuckle, but it was also a valid inquiry. It was not unusual for fatality review team members to become physically and emotionally uneasy when reviewing the intimate details of a death.

Vicarious trauma, or **secondary traumatic stress,** refers to emotional and psychological strain that results from continuous exposure to victims of trauma, including learning the details about their circumstances (McCann & Pearlman, 1990). Front-line workers who engage with populations who use drugs have reported high rates of secondary traumatic stress, which can lead to psychological duress and professional degradation (Wies et al., 2023). Vicarious trauma can impact one's body and mind similar to experiencing trauma first hand.

Some professionals have their own history of trauma, which attracted them to work with others in similar situations, but doing so could trigger memories and feelings that cause them to relive the trauma (Menschner & Maul, 2016).

The Office for Victims of Crime promotes a Vicarious Trauma Toolkit that includes suggestions for coworkers, supervisors, and family members of those experiencing vicarious trauma as they offer support to individuals: https://ovc.ojp.gov/program/vtt/introduction.

Self-care means taking time to do daily activities to improve physical and mental health. It is an important approach to preventing secondary trauma. Purposefully incorporating self-care is a strategy to help alleviate discouragement and emotional fatigue. More intense intervention (such as counseling) can help prevent professionals from becoming overwhelmed. As part of the program planning process, allocating time and resources for self-care is an important consideration.

Fabiola noted a national conference for the fatality review process that heavily promotes practicing self-care for team members – a type of technical and emotional roadmap for newer members of the team. She reflected, "It can be really hard to maintain energy to do this work when we review some really tragic cases, and the next month there's more of the same. Sometimes it can feel like the flow of cases is never-ending."

MAPPING A LIFE AND A DEATH THROUGH MULTIPLE SOURCES OF DATA

Several additional members joined the team after the first introductory meeting, including representatives from the city's public school district and the county coroner's office. The addition of new faces was a good sign – it meant that there were a variety of stakeholders who had vested interest in the endeavor. Furthermore, a strength of fatality review is that it taps into a wealth of personal and professional knowledge in one setting. Fabiola took on an educator's role when she said, "Diversity of team members is huge! Each member of the team enters into the process with a unique perspective. The more voices we have, the more we can conduct a holistic analysis and bring a multi-pronged approach toward prevention." Having representatives from medical, criminal justice, educational, social services, and other professional communities helped round out the investigation.

At the meeting, everyone at the U-shaped configuration of tables was invited to introduce themselves. They shared professional affiliations as well as personal motivations for engaging in this critical work. Many had worked in their field for extended periods of time and had a passion for helping prevent additional suffering in the community. A professor explained his desire to extend his potential influence outside the classroom and into the local community where he lived. And, as promised, there was food – sandwiches, salads, and pastries from a familiar franchise.

Fabiola distributed confidentiality forms to ensure that case-specific, sensitive information revealed would not leave the room. Identifying information about each case needed to be available so the team could check their own databases for useful details about a deceased person – details that could help the team understand how things could have happened differently if certain steps had been taken at key points in the person's life. The state had recently passed legislation granting fatality boards increased access to such information.

Confidentiality, or the release of private information, is an essential consideration when using data from existing records. The *Health Insurance Portability and Accountability Act of 1996* (referred to as HIPAA) mandates that healthcare providers must implement standards that protect and guard against the misuse of individually identifiable health information.

In some cases, data can be de-identified, meaning all information, including addresses, names, or other personal information, is removed from the record.

Fabiola presented a *PowerPoint* slide introducing the first case while team members flipped through a packet of reports containing background information about the overdose fatality victim. After taking a moment to read basic facts of the case – personal characteristics, marital and parental status, criminal and substance history, and employment status – group members consulted professional databases and found more information to throw into the mix:

- The coroner had investigated the scene of death at the victim's residence.
- The nurse provided context for substances found in the victim's body.
- The pharmacist commented on suspicious prescriptions.
- The police officer had met the victim's parents years ago when the victim was playing high school sports.

After nearly a half hour of exchanging information and probing for additional detail and insight, the facilitator shifted the focus of the discussion: "What could have been done to prevent this?"

> Prevention can occur on various levels.
> - **Primary prevention** includes efforts that prevent a disease, illness, or injury from ever occurring. Primary prevention aims to limit exposure to risk factors among a healthy population.
> - **Secondary prevention** includes efforts that lead to early diagnosis and prompt treatment of a disease, illness, or injury. Secondary prevention often means conducting screenings. It aims to minimize progression of a health problem.
> - **Tertiary prevention** includes efforts that prevent a disease, illness, or injury from getting worse. Tertiary prevention aims to reduce the severity of disease and is focused on rehabilitation.

Brainstorming ensued:

- Sufficient knowledge of warnings signals may have been lacking at school and home.
- The family may have been in denial of the seriousness of the situation.
- The victim had not faced serious consequences for prior misbehavior.
- The victim did not trust law enforcement or social workers.

These comments were not solutions as much as observations. Could the overdose victim have been aided in avoiding taking the first hit of a substance? If so, such efforts would be considered primary prevention. Could someone have detected the substance use and intervened early to help deter further misuse? If so, that would have been considered secondary prevention. Could better interventions have helped the individual sustain recovery from addiction? If so, that would be considered tertiary prevention. Being the first of many cases, it was difficult for the team members to connect the dots in a meaningful way, but eventually all the information and suggestions would be assembled into one master document to be analyzed for patterns that could inform future programming.

After reviewing two more cases, the anticipated fourth case review would wait until next time. The stories of human lives lost to substance misuse and suicide had taken their toll on the group – the mood was heavy. Grabbing an extra pastry on the way out might help a bit, but the serious work would pick up again in a month.

ANALYZING PATTERNS TO IDENTIFY FUTURE OPPORTUNITIES FOR INTERVENTION

When the 2020 pandemic arrived and social distancing became the norm, the fatality review process shifted to a videoconferencing medium. The transition was relatively smooth, and procedures otherwise mirrored the first case review meeting. The team viewed each *PowerPoint* slide through their electronic devices, listening to Fabiola elaborate on the details as her face appeared in the upper corner of the screen. Group members then consulted their professional databases or recalled their own clinical or legal interactions with the victim to add insight to the discussion.

Cases were often already familiar to team members. For example, one professional from the Department of Community Corrections mentioned the multiple times a person had the opportunity to engage in programming but chose not no; another professional had encounters with a person for 18 years, illustrating the numerous entry points for primary, secondary, and tertiary prevention. A representative of the Department of Child Services remembered that a victim had previously lived in a family investigated for child abuse and neglect.

The review process was no easier in this virtual format. The difficult realities of intergenerational trauma and addiction were still on display, and each member of the team did their best to avoid letting the heaviness dampen their desire to engage in the important work. However, with each new case reviewed, patterns started appearing that offered some hope for planning and designing future public health initiatives. For example, grief emerged as a common risk factor – several victims had lost family members and appeared to lack resources or capacity to work through the mourning process. One team member suggested to the group that hospitals could be key target points for helping family members find resources for confronting their grief after the passing of a loved one. Everyone was evaluating the data and putting their heads together to come up with future entry points for intervention.

Typically, after about 12–18 months, enough cases will have been reviewed to trigger a formal analysis of the accumulated data. In the team's case, given the interruptions due to the pandemic, the analysis began about two years after the initial meeting of the fatality review team. At that point, 18 cases had been reviewed by the county team and the group had made a total of 238 suggestions toward preventing suicides and overdoses. The Overdose Fatality Review Data Working Group, part of the state Department of Health's Division of Fatality Review and Prevention, analyzed the suggestions for common themes and offered three top recommendations for the county to consider in its future plans:

1. Strengthen follow-up efforts for those who miss substance use treatment;

2. Improve the referral process for connecting people to substance use and mental health treatment;

3. Increase prevention and treatment services aimed at youth.

The Overdose Fatality Review Data Working Group, consisting of professionals from the state Department of Health, the Centers for Disease Control, the Institute of Intergovernmental Research, and other representatives from other national institutes and state review boards, collect and process the data for each county. They look for patterns and trends related to the fatalities and assess the suggestions made by the county-level team. Results are shared with the county-level team who then makes recommendations about which next steps to prioritize and promote.

The Overdose Fatality Review Data Working Group promoted each recommendation and included strategies along with agencies that could help implement the recommendations. They shared a detailed report with the CCSUP that included background information on the 18 deceased individuals, along with the three main recommendations. It was also noted that, based on toxicology reports, opioids and fentanyl (a synthetic opioid) were the most common substances found in the systems of the deceased.

Fabiola summarized the next steps of the process, "Ideally, the next steps of this process include discussing recommendations with local leaders and organizational representatives who have the time, resources, and connections to be the change-makers in the community."

She chuckled, "We're going to have to convince some people to be the change makers we need." Such individuals or teams would write grants, plan and develop new programs, petition for policy changes, and guide local governments and agencies as to how to best use their resources to address fatality trends. Implemented recommendations would be monitored and assessed over time to evaluate their impact and to see if alterations needed to be made to enhance effectiveness. In the meantime, the fatality review team would continue to meet and study new cases, adding to the database for another review in a year or two.

Does all this work make a difference? Fabiola mentioned that these reviews can identify unanticipated patterns. She recalled a story from another county in the state where the overdose fatality review team was certain from the outset that their key problem was doctor and pharmacy shopping – individuals seeking out new opportunities to get duplicate opioid prescriptions to feed an addiction. However, it turned out that in 13 of the 14 overdose fatalities, the individual had only one doctor and one pharmacy. The county was thus able to focus their resources on other strategies more likely to prevent such fatalities. Another county discovered that most recent overdose fatalities happened to individuals who were divorced or going through a divorce. A mental health screening was consequently added to divorce court proceedings to guide people toward helpful services.

Nevertheless, evaluating the actual impact of fatality review teams – particularly by how many lives are saved – can be difficult (US Department of Health and Human Services Administration on Children Youth and Families Children's Bureau, 2012). Community fatalities can be caused by a complex set of factors, and linking fatality rates directly to the team's recommendations is complicated. Determining how many lives would not have been lost if the team had not implemented changes is also complicated. But, for this county team, while the process was just beginning, it had already revealed important insights that could help inform their future plans for prevention programs.

DISCUSSION QUESTIONS

1. What might be the advantages and disadvantages of using identifiable data for analysis?

2. How might bias be introduced when collecting different pieces of information? How can bias be mitigated?

3. Why is it beneficial to identify risk factors associated with the people you hope to help?

4. How do behavioral and environmental risk factors relate to one another?

5. What did you think about the idea of using obituaries and other information to remind team members of the person behind the data? How might it impact your program planning?

6. What did you notice about the need for team members to practice self-care? Have you ever felt the need for self-care? How have you met that need?

7. How could you build self-care into a program you plan?

8. Why might it be important to prioritize resources, or narrow a focus, when program planning?

9. In what ways might you plan in advance to have your program affect policy?

10. What does it mean that "where we chose to fix our attention would influence our outcome"? How can a group ensure that the intended purpose and scope of the review remains the same throughout the process?

11. Why should committees be composed of individuals who represent a variety of subgroups within the community?

ACTIVITY

1. Imagine you have an idea for a program that you are excited about and cannot wait to pitch to your state department of health. Discuss what you should do first to ensure that your idea will meet the needs of the community. What can you do to assess how well your program would fit within the community you hope to serve? In what ways might your program not be a good fit? How can you adapt your program to the needs you discover while maintaining enthusiasm for the program you originally had in mind?

REFERENCES

McCann, I. L. & Pearlman, L. A. (1990). Vicarious traumatization: A framework for understanding the psychological effects of working with victims. *Journal of Traumatic Stress*, 3(1), 131–149.

Menschner, C. & Alexandra Maul, A. (2016). *Key Ingredients for Successful Trauma-Informed Care Implementation*. Center for Health Care Strategies. https://www.samhsa.gov/sites/default/files/programs_campaigns/childrens_mental_health/atc-whitepaper-040616.pdf

U.S. Department of Health and Human Services Administration on Children Youth and Families Children's Bureau (2012). *Fatality Review Teams: A Literature Review.* https://wrma.com%2Fwp-content%2Fuploads%2F2014%2F10%2FLiterature-Review. pdf&usg=AOvVaw0957M2NxVLAb00K_kJRZOb

Wies, J., Place, J. M., & Placek, C. (2023). Understanding secondary traumatic stress among frontline healthcare workers in the opioid crisis. *Journal of Substance Use, epub.*

CHAPTER

3

MATERNAL TREATMENT PROGRAM

USING CONSUMER ANALYSIS TO TARGET A SPECIFIC SEGMENT OF THE POPULATION

In this chapter, staff members at a behavioral health center worked with a university researcher to conduct a grant-funded consumer analysis to better understand their patient population. In program planning, interventions should be considered on multiple levels of the socio-ecological model to address a population's needs.

Tucked in the corner of an otherwise nondescript community behavioral health center was a surprisingly bright room, lit up like a yellow and blue farmhouse, accented with a variety of cushioned gliders and rocking chairs. Those entering would need to step around baby changing stations, *Pack'n'Plays*, swings, bouncy chairs, and shape

Health Promotion Planning: Learning from the Accounts of Public Health Practitioners,
First Edition. Jean Marie S. Place, Jonel Thaller, and Scott S. Hall.
© 2024 John Wiley & Sons, Inc. Published 2024 by John Wiley & Sons, Inc.

sorters. Baby toys were strewn across plush carpeting and inspirational phrases filled the wall.

This colorful and welcoming room housed the behavioral health center's relatively new Maternal Treatment Program, situated within a specialized addictions and recovery division. The program's purpose was to provide therapeutic support for mothers struggling with addiction during and after pregnancy, including assistance with navigating Child Protective Services (CPS) if their children had been removed due to circumstances resulting from their addiction. Some of the women enrolled in the program had experienced high risk pregnancies or were tasked with caring for a medically fragile infant. Others had suffered infant loss during or after pregnancy. All had likely experienced significant trauma leading up to their time in the program. Some women who misuse substances, for example, have experienced childhood sexual abuse (Liebschutz et al., 2002).

Given women's traumatic histories, some experts recommend providing specialized services in women-only spaces and focusing on healing trauma as a pathway to sobriety. This approach of dividing a target population into groups of individuals with similar characteristics is an example of population segmentation. The Maternal Treatment Program had planned for gender-based segmentation, presuming it would increase the chances this population would respond positively to treatment services. Moreover, the Maternal Treatment Program referred to their service users as **consumers,** a term often used in the social service sector to refer to a "set of people who have an actual or potential interest in a product or service" (Kotler & Clarke, 1987, p. 108). Some programs choose to refer to their service users as "consumers" rather than "patients" or "clients" as a way to cultivate a consumer-centered culture of choice and empowerment. Empowerment was important to the program developers of the Maternal Treatment Program.

Segmentation allows program policies and delivery to be tailored to the common needs of a specific group. Experts suggest that segmenting consumers into smaller, meaningful subgroups can help guide which interventions may be most effective for different people (Figueroa, 2021).

Segmentation of a target population into more specific groups can be based on demographic factors such as gender, income, marital status, occupation, religion, race/ethnicity, and age. It can also be based on geographic factors, like zip code, or lifestyle factors, like interests and hobbies. Populations can be segmented based on readiness to change, knowledge, attitudes, or behaviors, as well as past experiences or complex health conditions (Engl et al., 2019).

USING THE SOCIAL-ECOLOGICAL FRAMEWORK TO UNDERSTAND BARRIERS AND FACILITATORS TO BEHAVIOR CHANGE

The Maternal Treatment Program had experienced many incredible successes during its first three years of operation, but there was one reoccurring and glaring issue: many women who were enrolled in the program were not regularly attending required therapeutic sessions. To address this problem, the program's director, Kate Fowler, invited a researcher from the local university, Dr. Ali Shaw, to help with a solution. Dr. Shaw came highly recommended as a program planning collaborator based on her work with programs in the community. She had earned a reputation as someone who put the needs of community members first before her need for status or clout. This was important to Kate, as she knew her staff would be somewhat suspicious of agency outsiders who claimed they could solve all the program's problems with research.

Kate cared deeply about her staff and the women served by the Maternal Treatment Program. She had worked hard to implement the program's intervention and wanted to ensure **program fidelity** – meaning that the program would be carried out as planned. Kate also hoped to achieve a sufficient **program reach** – allowing many women the opportunity to participate – and to have a strong **program response** – with women following through with participation. For this program, regular attendance was especially important because clinicians would assess the women's improvement according to their adherence to the structured curriculum. Thus, the success of the program would be based upon the women's level of improvement and on the number of women served. Kate knew that the Maternal Treatment Program risked losing future funding if the number of women regularly attending sessions fell short of the program's predetermined goals.

Fidelity refers to when programs are implemented according to plan and follow established protocols. If a program is implemented as intended, researchers can appropriately assess whether the program influenced outcomes. However, if a program is implemented poorly, it is unclear whether a lack of desirable outcomes is due to poor implementation of the program or to the effectiveness of the program itself.

Carroll et al. (2007) proposed a framework for addressing fidelity:

- Assess participant adherence to the program, including whether the intervention was received by the participants as often and for as long as it should have been.
- Consider whether factors have affected the delivery process, including facilitation strategies, quality of delivery, and participant responsiveness.

During her first face-to-face meeting with Dr. Shaw, Kate sank into one of the plush gliding chairs as she described her concerns about the future of the program. She hoped that Dr. Shaw could help her brainstorm ways to increase attendance among the target population. While some women were court-ordered to attend services at the Maternal Treatment Program, others arrived there voluntarily. But the challenge of arriving – much less arriving on time – was a collision course of transportation issues, morning sickness, and childcare needs. Many program participants were lost to attrition and subsequent relapse. To increase participation, Kate had tried to implement an incentive system. As she recalled this effort, she motioned to a row of closets, well-stocked with new and gently used baby clothes and toys that women could purchase with points earned for regular attendance. But, she noted, the well-intended incentive system was not working.

Leaning back into their padded rockers, Kate and Dr. Shaw contemplated the situation together. They both wanted to know more about what led women to the treatment center and why they did not follow through with attending sessions. What was missing? Were they doing enough? How could they better attract and retain women who needed services? Kate was confronting a sobering reality: segmentation might not be enough to meet these women's recovery needs. But what were the women's needs? Kate felt that she and her staff had built trust and rapport with most of the program's consumers, yet many still struggled with attendance. Dr. Shaw acknowledged Kate's frustrations but reminded her that data could help elucidate the women's barriers to attendance and what they might need to respond to treatment more positively.

Dr. Shaw emphasized the importance of identifying barriers and facilitators to accessing services like the Maternal Treatment Program to evaluate what was working for women in the program and what was working against them. Did women have the resources they needed to help them thrive, such as strong social support, problem-solving skills, positive role models, and steady housing? Such factors bolster a woman's capacity to steer away from risks, withstand triggers, and overcome stress. When seeking services, do women face discrimination, stigma, excessive costs, or breaches of privacy? Women with facilitative factors, such as safe housing, reliable transportation, and health insurance, were more likely to be successful in recovery than women with double shifts, high rent, low self-confidence, and no transportation. Kate needed to better understand the worlds in which the women lived so that the Maternal Treatment Program could be adapted to better meet their needs. The objective was to protect and promote women's recovery by creating an environment specific to their needs.

Barriers prevent people from engaging in a service and impede behavior change.

Facilitators promote engaging in a service and aid in behavior change.

The **social-ecological framework** is a useful way to understand the barriers and facilitators of individuals' health behaviors. This framework was originally developed to understand the multiple dimensions that influence a person's health (McLeroy et al., 1988; Stokols, 1996). Looking beyond individual factors, like heredity or biology, the social-ecological approach encourages understanding of a person's relationships, the community in which they live, and other organizational or structural influences. The framework aims to describe the relationship between humans and their physical and social environments, recognizing that external relationships and environments have an impact on a person's health.

Dr. Shaw was convinced that a consumer analysis was needed to uncover the wants, needs, and preferences of the target population, as well as the barriers and facilitators to behavior change. With this data, they could determine why women were not meeting program attendance requirements and then determine a strategy to address the women's unmet needs.

Sitting amongst so many colorful baby toys, Dr. Shaw suggested that they seek grant funding to move forward with conducting the analysis. A grant application would require them to outline a plan that included detailed goals, expectations, and day-to-day operations within the parameters of limited money, time, and personnel. They needed to craft this plan upfront before any data collection took place.

Grants are a useful way to bring external funding to an organization, which can be used for a variety of purposes, including acquiring equipment and/or supplies, hiring staff, purchasing curriculum, launching new programs, or conducting research. Grants are often offered by state and federal governments, foundations, or research centers.

A *request for proposal* (RFP) issued by a funder will outline what applicants need to submit to be considered for funding. Grant funders often require the following information when considering whether an effort is worth financing:

- Researcher qualifications and experience
- The general problem or need

■ Anticipated outcomes

■ Activities to be undertaken

■ Timeline

■ Evaluation measures

■ Budget

A large part of a consumer analysis is asking consumers directly about their wants and needs. Dr. Shaw knew they needed to collect data from among the target population – pregnant and postpartum women with substance use disorders – but how? What methods would be most appropriate, effective, and affordable? Should they ask women to fill out a closed-ended survey about their wants, needs, and preferences? This would be considered a **quantitative method** where a survey or questionnaire would offer standardized responses for the participants to choose from. Or, should Dr. Shaw interview women face-to-face to discuss in-depth what influenced their drug misuse, addressing both the personal (e.g. Can you talk about the role of your friends? Did you have family members who used drugs?) and the broader considerations (e.g. Were you able to access annual check-ups with a healthcare provider?). This approach would be considered a **qualitative method** where an interview comprised of open-ended questions would allow respondents to answer freely using their own words.

Dr. Shaw considered the logistics of recruiting women to take part in the research. Where would they find specific women who were misusing opioids or other illicit substances? Considering the stigma attached to maternal drug use, or even drug use in general, how could they convince the women that their confidentiality would be maintained?

Indeed, finding women to participate in the consumer analysis ended up being a significant challenge for Dr. Shaw. Women with substance use disorders are a "hard-to-reach" population, meaning "sub-groups of the population that are difficult to reach or involve in research or public health programs due to their physical and geographical location or their social and economic situation" (Shaghaghi et al., 2011). Drug use is a social situation that could lead to criminalization, incarceration, or unwanted exposure and stigma, so it is not hard to imagine why some women would not want to participate in a research study. Dr. Shaw noted that many women were too scared to come forward and participate because they were afraid they would be reported to CPS.

Doing research, whether grant-funded or not, generally requires obtaining *Institutional Review Board (IRB)* approval. The IRB is responsible for reviewing a research plan before implementation to ensure it is ethical and free of coercion.

If the research involves human subjects, like interviewing people or collecting data through surveys, the IRB will review an **informed consent document**, which communicates any potential risks of the research to the participants, including mental anguish or breach of confidentiality.

The IRB will also review advertisements or other methods used to recruit participants. The IRB will pay special attention to groups of potential participants considered a "protected population" such as pregnant people, students, and children.

To conduct the consumer analysis, Dr. Shaw planned to contact as many pregnant and postpartum women as possible, knowing that she could filter and find those who misuse substances among the women she contacted. The goal was to contact at least 200 women.

She decided to use structured, quantitative surveys to understand women's social-economic status, their employment history, the number of adverse childhood experiences (ACEs) they had experienced (ACEs can predict long-term health outcomes like substance misuse), and other numeric information that could provide insight into the barriers or facilitators of women's participation in services. As part of the research, and after participants had consented to the procedure, she would also ask women for a saliva sample to assess the presence or absence of substances in their system. For this research, she was interested in the few tests that would come back with double lines – the positive tests.

Through this process, it was important to identify and establish relationships with **key stakeholders** – people, communities, and organizations with a vested interest in the results of the research. The stakeholders for this study included CEOs, executive directors, and chief physicians of medical centers whose job it was to deliver effective services to the target population. These stakeholders would play a crucial role in the research by allowing Dr. Shaw and her team to enter their facilities to recruit participants. For this reason, some stakeholders are also referred to as **gatekeepers**, as their figurative stamp of approval can make or break whether researchers gain access to potential study participants. Ideally, a mutually beneficial relationship is forged between the research team and stakeholders.

Dr. Shaw needed to get the stakeholders excited about the research process and clearly communicate how the results of the consumer analysis could inform future interventions, making it easier for women to access the services they need (Frew et al., 2014). She reached out to a contact she knew at a local health center, which provided services to low-income clients in the community. She met with Daniel, a friendly CEO with a kind blue eyes and prematurely graying hair. Daniel enthusiastically agreed to let Dr. Shaw use the community health center facility for study recruitment. They agreed that, with IRB approval, the research team would post study recruitment flyers in waiting room areas and bathrooms. Dr. Shaw was not shy about putting flyers into the hands of physicians and receptionists, too. She hoped to build a more human connection with stakeholders with her physical presence and surmised that giving them some responsibility for sharing the flyers with prospective participants would keep the study at the forefront of their minds.

Daniel, the likeable CEO, opened the center's doors to Dr. Shaw and her research team, but whether women who misuse opioids would want to participate in the research, or front office staff would be supportive of the study, remained to be seen. Armed with clipboards, flyers, and audio recorders, undergraduate university students were hired to help collect data at the health center. Though eager and excited, they often sat for two-hour stretches without administering a single survey. Receptionists who had agreed to help by sharing flyers at the check-in desks simply waved on women to their perinatal care appointments without any mention of the study. With some frustration, Dr. Shaw noted, "The people working the front desk always acted like they didn't know what was going on." The frontline staff may not have understood the purpose of the study, were overworked, or were simply not invested in the research. Either way, Dr. Shaw and her research team did not make much progress.

After several months and only 16 successful interviews, data collection stalled at the health center. Dr. Shaw reasoned, "I couldn't keep pushing for something when, obviously, I think this was their way of saying, 'We're not interested.'" She tried similar recruitment strategies at two other health centers in town with a modest yield of several more participants.

Looking back on the research process, Dr. Shaw noted that establishing a Memorandum of Understanding (MOU), or formal written agreement with the health centers about their participation in the research, might have helped everyone to commit to a data collection schedule and protocol.

Pre-planning helps stakeholders avoid confusion in the implementation process. Pre-planning ensures all stakeholders are aware of the purpose of the project, understand the scope and timeframe, have a solid idea of the anticipated outcomes, agree to their roles and responsibilities, and understand what is expected of them. Collaboration on a **memorandum of understanding (MOU)** to outline responsibilities and use of resources (McKenzie et al., 2017) facilitates project "buy-in" and ensures that all parties – including the researchers – understand expectations about the length of the study, the type of work involved, and who is responsible for oversight (Placek et al., 2021).

Dr. Shaw cast an even wider net of recruitment by moving beyond the health centers to various community venues. She ran digital advertisements at the local university, distributed flyers at the downtown library, spoke with local breastfeeding groups, and posted on "mommy-&-me" social media sites. These additional recruitment tactics resulted in 24 more pregnant women participating in the study, but only one from this group had misused substances and could truly be considered part of the target population.

The research team also engaged in a tactic referred to as **snowball recruitment**, which is when study participants are encouraged to refer other eligible participants. Participants who successfully recruited more eligible women to participate in the study received a $5 gift card in addition to their original $15 compensation, but unfortunately, this method did not generate any additional participants.

In the original grant application, the researchers proposed that data would be collected from over 200 women. However, over the course of one and a half years, Dr. Shaw and her team collected only 23 completed surveys. They were blindsided by the difficulty of collecting data on this "hard to reach" population.

A WAY FORWARD BASED ON CONSUMER PREFERENCES

Ultimately, Dr. Shaw and her research team returned from community-based recruitment back to the door of the Maternal Treatment Center. They were trying to understand perspectives of women misusing drugs – both those in treatment and those not in treatment – to understand broad perspectives of barriers and facilitators for seeking health services. Dr. Shaw reflected:

When you do not know who the population is that struggles most with addiction, there has to be some openness in your methods. You have to allow anyone to join, who falls within the pregnant postpartum criteria, and then you just have to get creative on how to access women from different pockets of the community.

Once again, seated in the plush rocking chairs, Dr. Shaw asked Kate if she could contact women attending the program – but this time she asked if she could also sit down with women to conduct qualitative, in-depth interviews. She was able to supplement the low survey recruitment with 10 in-depth qualitative interviews with women attending the Maternal Treatment Program. It was in these intimate, private settings that she learned the richest lessons on barriers across the social–ecological framework that impeded successful recovery from addiction.

The Centers for Disease Control (CDC, 2022) categorized risk and protective factors that affect health, grounded in the social-ecological framework:

- The individual or intrapersonal level includes biology and other personal characteristics like age, education, income, and health history. It also includes attitudes, beliefs, knowledge, and behaviors.
- The interpersonal level includes relationships within a social circle, such as friends, partners, and family members.
- The organizational or institutional level includes the settings in which people operate, such as schools, healthcare centers, workplaces, businesses, and faith-based organizations. It considers the characteristics of those settings that may influence health.
- The community level is focused on the relationships between organizations and institutions and includes the built environment of neighborhoods and surroundings.
- The societal level looks at broad societal factors, such as cultural and social norms and health, economic, educational, and social laws and policies on national and local levels.

Ultimately, Dr. Shaw was pleased with the qualitative data collected for the consumer analysis because she was able to meet the treatment program's original goal, which was to learn more about barriers and facilitators for program participation. She heard many impactful stories while sitting across from women. The conversations occurred in the same room where Dr. Shaw sat across from Kate, the program director. She reflected, "It seems as though most women who are recovering from substance addiction are also recovering from life-long trauma and the pain that triggered the addiction." She related how important it is for others to understand "the trajectory of pain that they've experienced throughout their lives and how hard it is to make a huge shift away from addiction at such a critical time point in life."

Through her research, Dr. Shaw identified the following barriers that pregnant and postpartum women experienced in their journey to recovery, situated within the social-ecological framework:

- On an individual level, many women discussed the difficulty of overcoming early childhood trauma. For many women, sexual trauma was a part of their childhoods, which is consistent with research findings that up to 81% of women with substance use disorders experienced some form of sexual or physical abuse (Liebschutz et al., 2002).
- On an interpersonal level, one woman talked about how her co-workers used substances at work and the abundance of drug use in schools. Being surrounded by other people who use substances, including close family members, was a significant challenge to sobriety.
- On an organizational level, women discussed the role of CPS. It was often mentioned as a system that worked against mothers (e.g. "I know I relapsed because I had my daughter taken."). Women reflected on how punitive it felt to have children removed, some-times causing them to sink into a depressive state. Removing children can be a necessary step to recovery, but women discussed how the Department of Child Services as an organization felt threatening rather than supportive.
- On a community level, transportation was consistently mentioned as a barrier. The location of the Maternal Treatment Program on the north side of town, as opposed to the south side where many participants lived, made traveling to sessions three times a week notably difficult. The lack of bus stops, the frigid winter weather, and the challenge of arriving on time were identified as community barriers.
- Finally, on a societal level, overall stigma against people who misuse substances was a strong and painful barrier. One woman stated, "I think [stigma] is such a strong barrier to treatment because it feels like the community doesn't believe in your ability to succeed. I wish they could let go of the attitude that 'once an addict always an addict.'"

Dr. Shaw asked the women about supportive, facilitative factors that helped them seek out and attend treatment. Taking on the perspective of the consumer – or having a consumer orientation – can help planners and practitioners see the program through different eyes. The women discussed what they liked about the program:

- The women liked that the program offered peer support where women could learn from others who were experiencing similar problems.
- They were deeply grateful that children were allowed to come to sessions, although it was still painful for those women whose children had been removed by CPS.
- They appreciated that, unlike Narcotics Anonymous, services could be private and individualized.
- They expressed value at having access to a nonjudgmental, empathetic healthcare provider.

Consumer orientation "is a dedicated effort to understand the priority population prior to developing an intervention and then keeping knowledge of the target population at the center of all program planning decisions" (Mckenzie et al., 2017).

Almost all the women she interviewed rallied around one suggestion: Neighborhood-based treatment. They wanted to receive help in the context of their own familiar neighborhood. This insight was critical because of the concept of competition. Competition is the idea that people can choose between positive or negative behaviors. To promote a positive behavior like attending sessions at the Maternal Treatment Program, instead of a competing behavior, like staying in bed or consuming drugs, planners need to make it as easy as possible for people to perform the desired behavior. The women's input compelled the staff members at the Maternal Treatment Program to consider how challenging it was for women to attend sessions because of the schedule and location of services. Kate and her staff were motivated to create a better way. They considered the following:

- What would make it easy for the target population to obtain treatment services? Women consistently reported the desire for treatment to be closer to where they lived and worked.
- What made it difficult for the target population to attend services regularly? Women talked about sleeping through early morning alarm clocks due to late nights with fussy babies or missed buses

that set their schedule back until the next bus was available. Any delay with childcare could throw the whole day into disarray.

- What benefit did the target population want as a result of going to treatment? They wanted to get better faster. In other words, they wanted treatment that aggressively addressed withdrawal symptoms and a management approach that included medication assisted treatment (Davis et al., 2021). They also wanted treatment to increase access to and connection with their children.

- What type of program would the target population participate in? They indicated strong interest in treatment programs that combine medication assisted treatment with counseling. This is aligned with Davis et al. (2021) who found cognitive behavioral approaches were particularly helpful for women.

- Where did the target population want the services offered? Women said they wanted treatment options available in their neighborhoods.

- At what time of the day would the target population like the services offered? Women suggested that evening hours should be offered, as well as daytime hours, to accommodate varying work schedules.

- What was the best way to communicate information to the target population about the services? Women urged their community to break the stigma of the "shitty, drugged-up parent" and to consider ways to talk about services that were not stigmatizing.

Ultimately, as a result of the data collection process, Dr. Shaw and her research team proposed a mobile treatment unit that could be stationed in the southern part of the city, far more accessible than where the current treatment center was located. A mobile unit, similar to a fully equipped recreational vehicle with a private, medical treatment area, as well as a waiting room, could help women overcome barriers identified in the consumer analysis. Dr. Shaw had considered what she learned about the target population and their preferences to make this strategic recommendation.

Dr. Shaw collaborated with Kate and other staff members of the Maternal Treatment Program to prepare another grant proposal to bring a mobile treatment unit to the south side neighborhoods. Dr. Shaw concluded, "If we're using the social-ecological model to understand pathways to addiction and why women stay in recovery, then, obviously, we need a treatment program that addresses these levels."

DISCUSSION QUESTIONS

1. What are some advantages and disadvantages of focusing a program on a single, specific segment of consumers?

2. Can you think of examples of segmented services in your own community?

3. What resources or strategies can you think of that could help recruit "hard to reach" populations?

4. What barriers can you think of that could prevent people from completing a program? How can you plan for addressing such barriers ahead of time?

5. If you were the member of a target population and were being recruited into a study, how much money would you find to be an effective incentive for your participation? In this chapter, the researchers offered a $5 gift card to incentivize recruiting more participants. Do you think this amount is a sufficient incentive? Why or why not?

6. What are the ethical implications of providing monetary incentives to participate in research studies to people who use drugs? What other incentives might a researcher offer?

7. What are other individual, interpersonal, organizational, community and societal level barriers to recovery from addiction beyond what is mentioned in this chapter?

8. Why was attendance at the program so important to the staff? What is the potential impact of lack of attendance on program fidelity?

9. Why was a grant application an important part of the research process? In what ways can grant funding contribute to the research process?

ACTIVITIES

1. Imagine you are seeking funding for a consumer analysis so you can learn the interests of potential consumers related to a new program. However, such consumers are part of a "hard to reach population." In about 250–300 words, write a portion of a grant proposal that describes (1) the concept of "hard to reach population," (2) challenges to recruiting this population, and (3) the importance of having financial incentives to attract this population. Share your writing in small groups and work to come up with one single writing that uses the best of each other's contributions.

   ▪ Distinct "hard to reach populations" could be assigned to each student group, such as:

> ▪ the homeless and transient, chronically mentally ill, young people who drop-out of high school, criminal offenders, sex workers, justice-involved youth, gang members, and unhoused youth (Lambert & Wiebel, 1990).

2. Based on the scenario in the chapter, groups of students can role play the process of creating a memorandum of understanding (MOU). Roles can include the agency that hosts the program, the researchers who lead the study, the university that provides that student research assistants, and the health center who assists with recruitment. Students can look for examples of MOUs online, or use a free service such as rocketlawyer.com to create one.

REFERENCES

Carroll, C., Patterson, M., Wood, S., Booth, A., Rick, J., & Balain, S. (2007). A conceptual framework for implementation fidelity. *Implementation Science*, 2(40). https://implementationscience.biomedcentral.com/articles/10.1186/1748-5908-2-40

CDC (2022). *The Social-Ecological Model: A Framework for Prevention.* https://www.cdc.gov/violenceprevention/about/social-ecologicalmodel.html

Davis, J. P., Eddie, D., Prindle, J., Dworkin, E. R., Christie, N. C., Saba, S., . . . & Kelly, J. F. (2021). Sex differences in factors predicting post-treatment opioid use. *Addiction*, *116*(8), 2116–2126.

Engl, E., Smittenaar, P., & Sgaier, S. K. (2019). Identifying population segments for effective intervention design and targeting using unsupervised machine learning: An end-to-end guide. *Gates Open Research*, *3*(2). https://doi.org/10.12688/gatesopenres.13029.2

Figueroa, J. (2021). High-need, high-cost segmentation framework. https://www.bettercareplaybook.org/resources/high-need-high-cost-segmentation-framework

Frew, P. M., Saint-Victor, D. S., Isaacs, M. B., Kim, S., Swamy, G. K., Sheffield, J. S., & Ault, K. (2014). Recruitment and retention of pregnant women into clinical research trials: An overview of challenges, facilitators, and best practices. *Clinical Infectious Diseases: An Official Publication of the Infectious Diseases Society of America*, *59*(Suppl 7), S400–S407. https://doi.org/10.1093/cid/ciu726.

Kotler, P. & Clarke, R. (1987). *Marketing for Health Care Organizations*. Englewood Cliffs, NJ: Prentice Hall.

Lambert E. Y. & Wiebel, W. W., editor (1990). *The Collection and Interpretation of Data from Hidden Populations*. Washington, DC: United States National Institute on Drug Abuse. http://www.drugabuse.gov/pdf/monographs/download98.html.

Liebschutz, J., Savetsky, J. B., Saitz, R., Horton, N. J., Lloyd-Travaglini, C., & Samet, J. H. (2002). The relationship between sexual and physical abuse and substance abuse consequences. *Journal of Substance Abuse Treatment*, *22*(3), 121–128.

McKenzie, J., Neiger, B., & Thackeray, R. (2017). *Planning, Implementing, and Evaluating Health Promotion Programs* (7th ed.). USA: Pearson.

McLeroy, K. R., Bibeau, D., Steckler, A., & Glanz, K. (1988). An ecological perspective on health promotion programs. *Health Education Quarterly*, 15(4), 351–377.

Placek, C. D., Place, J. M., & Wies, J. (2021). Reflections and challenges of pregnant and post-partum participant recruitment in the context of the opioid epidemic. *Maternal and Child Health Journal. 25*(7), 1031–1035.

Shaghaghi, A., Bhopal, R. S., & Sheikh, A. (2011). Approaches to recruiting 'hard-to-reach'populations into research: a review of the literature. *Health Promotion Perspectives, 1*(2), 86.

Stokols, D. (1996). Translating social ecological theory into guidelines for community health promotion. *American Journal of Health Promotion, 10*(4), 282–298.

CHAPTER

RECOVERY
RIDE AND RALLY

EVENT PLANNING AND PROCESS
IMPROVEMENT

In this chapter, we show you a "behind the scenes" look at an event planner who worked to bring awareness to substance use disorder and promote recovery. The logistical details of organizing, implementing, and evaluating health promotion events are critical components to program planning.

On a Saturday morning in a public park in a bustling downtown, a woman stood under the canopy of a mobile cart and a glossy sign branded with the logo, *Sober Joe Coffee Co.*

"I'd like some coffee. What's good?"

The friendly, middle-aged man behind the makeshift counter was well-versed in the product and pointed to a list of coffees behind him, indicating which were available.

"Today we have our *Seize the Day* blend hot and the *Dark Before Dawn* on cold drip."

He enthusiastically launched into a description of how the cold-drip was made – from fair-trade coffee and in his own kitchen. He finished describing the process, then added, "Every cup you buy provides financial support for recovery agencies." The woman plunked an extra dollar in the donation jar next to the register. Several copies of the Big Book, the "bible" of Alcoholics Anonymous (AA), were also near the register, fanned out on the counter for any passer-by who desired one.

The *Sober Joe Coffee Co.* booth was one of many set up in the park that day in preparation for a public celebration of sobriety, the 15th annual Recovery Ride and Rally, funded by the state's Mental Health America and organized by one of its subsidiaries, the Addiction Issues Coalition. The stage and various booths were still being set up, and a spirit of celebration and camaraderie hung in the air. It was a beautiful September morning, and the park was quickly filling with people dressed primarily in purple or white t-shirts. Purple is the color of recovery and September is recovery month. Purple connotes wisdom, enlightenment, and pride (Mohebbi, 2014), and it was undeniable that people at the Recovery Ride and Rally felt a healthy dose of all three.

Three people in purple t-shirts smiled and posed for a photo with a large banner that read "We Are Recovery." The front of the purple shirts said, "I am one of 'THOSE' People!" and on the back, "We Do Recover" with a weblink to the Addictions Issue Coalition's home page. The white shirts read simply, "Sober AF." More purple and white t-shirts were neatly stacked on a table nearby with a line of people waiting to retrieve them. Some were picking up shirts they had prepaid for through Internet registration or earned by volunteering at the event, and others were buying shirts at the table for $15 each.

According to industry experts, selling t-shirts and other merchandise is a good idea for events like these (Penney, 2018). Not only can it increase awareness of the event, but it is also a way to raise money – a serious win for the event planners who earn money *and* get ongoing advertising through the person who bought the t-shirt and proudly wears it.

As more bodies began to populate the park, the opening musical act spilled onto the stage. The band began tuning instruments and testing microphones. A small crowd gathered around them in anticipation, though most attendees were still preparing for the recovery walk or circling around the exhibition area, looking over materials, collecting agency swag, and talking to people in or around the booths. Many seemed to know one another and shared warm greetings and side hugs.

DIVERSE SOURCES OF FUNDING ARE CRITICAL TO THE SUSTAINABILITY OF THE EVENT

The people at this lively event had come together for a very specific reason: to celebrate recovery from addiction. According to the event organizer, Juli Kohl, Deputy Director of the Addictions Issues Coalition, the Recovery Ride and Rally began 15 years ago as a casual grassroots celebration that included a motorcycle ride followed by a picnic in a much smaller park. At that time, the event was simply called the Recovery Ride. Why a motorcycle ride? The director of the Addictions Issue Coalition at the time was a biker.

Juli, a person in long-term recovery, became involved in organizing the Recovery Ride and Rally four years prior when she joined the Board of the Addictions Issues Coalition. She was put in charge of the event two years later when she stepped down from the board and became the Deputy Director.

Juli's predecessor, Sue Hunter, no longer worked at the Addictions Issues Coalition, but Juli had access to Sue's planning files from past years and could count on her to continue organizing the motorcycle portion of the event, which she described as "a well-oiled machine." Juli noted that, because it costs money to hire police escorts, "there's been talk with the board about whether we should continue the motorcycle ride, but there's so many people that have done it for several years from the beginning, so I love keeping that real." This year, they were fortunate that an officer volunteered to escort the riders out of Southside Harley, so it was not an expenditure. Additionally, Juli added that Sue set up a tent at the start of the ride each year and provided the riders, usually about 50 in total, with coffee and donuts donated by Southside Harley. She noted, "Sue has a really good system, and I felt it was important to keep that intact."

There are several ways to finance health promotion programs.

- **In-kind support** are contributions in the form of materials, labor, training, space, and/or access to networking connections. They are nonmonetary items that are voluntarily given without expectation of compensation in return.

- **Participant fees** require people to pay an amount to engage in a program. Participant fees can simply offset the cost of a program or contribute to a profit. They can serve the function of motivating participants to commit to attending the program, referred to as **ownership**. The obvious disadvantage of participant fees is that they could discourage participation among populations unable to pay.

- **Event sponsorship** is when an organization pays a fee or provides funding in exchange for promotional opportunities and brand exposure.
- **Third-party support** means that outside agencies help cover a portion of the program's costs. An organization other than the program planners or the participants themselves may pay for the program, such as an insurance company, civic group, professional association, or employer. Sometimes a combination of participant fee and third-party support is used, known as *cost sharing*. In some cases, participants are asked to pay a fee upfront, and upon completion of a program, may be reimbursed by a third party.

The Addictions Issues Coalition organized the rally and received funding support from the state's Mental Health America, who in turn, received funding from the federal Substance Abuse and Mental Health Administration (SAMHSA), under the US Department of Health and Human Services. Thus, tax dollars were used, in part, to fund the event. Admission to the event had always been free, but in the past two years, under Juli's leadership, the event started to raise money from the sale of t-shirts, rental fees for vendor and exhibition booths, corporate and nonprofit sponsorships, and optional paid registration for the recovery ride or walk.

When Juli solicited vendors to participate in the rally for the first time, she anticipated that perhaps 10 or so would want to be involved, but nearly 30 signed up. All paid a fee to set up their booths ($100 for nonprofits and $200 for for-profits), an amount that was decided upon with the help of more experienced fundraising specialists at Mental Health America.

The event also received sponsorships from Walmart, the state's flagship university, and for-profit treatment centers, among others. The logos of the sponsors, depending on their level of sponsorship, were displayed on marketing materials and banners at the event. General admission to the event was still free, but individuals could donate $15 to participate in the walk or ride ($40 for families). This year, 50 riders and 84 walkers were registered, and all who registered received a #WeAreRecovery bag and bandana.

Juli and the board did not have a specific fundraising goal in mind when they started, but she noted, "We definitely surpassed our expectations and came out ahead. We kind of had an idea going into it, but we were pleasantly surprised." The money earned from the fundraising went back into the general funds of the state's Mental Health America and the Addictions Issues Coalition to support the expansion of peer recovery programs.

Relying on fundraising requires knowing how to effectively understand and approach potential donors. The following tips are worth considering (Clepper, 2023):

- Know your donors – be sure to have correct contact information and understand the interests and histories of potential donors so you know best how to contact them and how to ask in a way that appeals to their goals.

- Prioritize stewardship – build lasting relationships with donors by sharing information about the impact their donations have and showing appreciation for their involvement.

- Target small donors – having many donors with modest donations is more stable than relying on a few large donors who could discontinue support.

- Consider corporate partnerships – local businesses can sponsor events or help you get connected with other potential sponsors through their community connections.

- Cultivate relationships with local press – do more than just send media requests to help draw attention to your cause; build relationships so that media professionals become motivated to spread the word.

- Highlight stories – share specific, moving examples of how your program has made a difference in people's lives; stories are powerful, especially when they include images.

- Make it simple to donate – provide suggested donation amounts, offer several payment methods, use QR codes; anticipate what complicates the donation process and make is simpler.

- Be straight forward and concise – be respectful of people's time by directly asking for donations while keeping information brief (though sufficiently detailed); be sure donors know what you are asking for and why.

For the first time, the rally moved to a larger park to accommodate the activities and the anticipation of more attendees. The event spanned nearly an entire day, from 10:30 a.m. to 3 p.m., with a roster full of activities: the motorcycle ride, a recovery walk, multiple acts of live musical entertainment, inspirational speakers, and children's activities that included face paint and purple cotton candy.

THE SUCCESS OF THE EVENT REQUIRES CAREFUL PLANNING AND COLLABORATION WITH PARTNERS

Despite its recent expansion, Juli indicated that the Recovery Ride and Rally lacked an official planning committee. The Recovery Ride and

Rally began organically within the recovery community as a small, informal event. An official planning committee was never part of the process.

> The purpose of a **planning committee**, sometimes referred to as a *steering committee* or *advisory board*, is not only to delegate tasks to helpers who may be best suited to completing them but also to adopt a more deliberate and comprehensive approach to planning, such as integrating fundraising into activities, strengthening partnerships with external stakeholders, or ensuring the event aligns with the organization's strategic plan.
>
> The size of an ideal planning committee depends on the event or program, but it should generally be large enough to accomplish the planning tasks and small enough that decision-making and involvement does not become cumbersome. If a committee becomes too large, subcommittees can be designated for specific tasks.
>
> A planning committee should include members of the target population, sometimes referred to as the priority population, to cultivate program ownership. Planners should ensure their voice is included at every stage of planning.
>
> Further, when developing a planning committee, it is helpful to consider the role of doers versus influencers. The **doers** are people who fully engage in the work and produce dependable deliverables. The **influencers**, who are just as crucial, are members who hold notable social, economic, or political power within the community. Their endorsement facilitates program success, and they can sometimes move program goals forward simply by making a phone call or sending an email.
>
> Depending on the circumstance, planning committee members can be chosen by invitation, election, appointment, or application. A **chairperson** should also be designated to lead the committee.

During her involvement, Juli recalled that most planning decisions were made informally by any member of the board who cared to be involved in the planning process. Juli had maintained this structure moving forward, preserving the most basic elements of the event but adding new features, like fundraising, with the support of board members. In addition to consulting the board, she said most major decisions about the event happened in informal conversation with the Director of the Addiction Issues Coalition, who works in the office next to hers. Ultimately, she says that she would like to have more people involved in planning, to meet on at least a monthly basis.

According to Juli, the current planning process for the event leveraged much of the operational infrastructure already provided by Mental Health America – a type of cooperative agreement. Mental Health America lended their marketing and IT staff to the event to develop advertising materials and a website for registration, donations, and sponsorship. Additionally, a Mental Health America grant writer helped Juli with sponsorship forms, making sure they were worded properly. Juli explained that it was helpful to have experts from Mental Health America oversee her planning tasks because she had to make sure certain components of marketing, such as use of logos, met the guidelines of the organization. Once the marketing materials and website were created, Mental Health America sent out advertising for the event through their statewide listserv of over 6,000 contacts, in addition to "word-of-mouth and people spreading the word through their own communities," Juli noted.

Cooperative agreements establish that two parties will mutually support each other through the exchange of resources in offering a program or service. Cooperative agreements are sometimes formalized in a document called **a memorandum of understanding (MOU)** or *memorandum of agreement (MOA)*.

Juli also sought help from outside sources she knew would be interested in helping, including her colleague and friend Becky. Juli explained, "You want Becky on your team with any event you're planning. She's very good at rallying troops." Becky was instrumental in drumming up volunteers for the day of the event, though Juli added that recruiting help for the event within the recovery community often happened organically because people in recovery were typically excited for an opportunity to celebrate their successes. She explained, "They want to share." Utilizing members of the recovery community as volunteers or, better yet, as members of a formal planning committee is important because, as the target population, they have a perspective that may differ from that of other professionals.

On the morning of the event, volunteers recruited mostly from residential recovery programs showed up in masse to help set up where needed. They earned a free t-shirt and could help themselves to donuts, but Juli recalled that many seemed happy just to be a part of the process. "They showed up early to set up our tables, and they kept coming up to me and saying, 'Where do you need me now? What can I do?'" At one end of the venue, volunteers set up a registration booth where attendees who had preregistered could pick up a bag and bandanna, both purple and emblazoned with #WeAreRecovery.

With so many moving parts, Juli reported that she was planning the event for probably six to eight months prior to its occurrence: "It's definitely an event that you need to plan year-round." Immediately after one year's event, she began to determine a date for the next year. She needed to make sure that the venue would be available again and would not conflict with any other popular events in the city. According to Juli, setting the date is the first step in the planning process, then securing the venue, then reaching out to sponsors, vendors, and exhibitors to make sure they have time to work the fees into their budgets.

Juli said she had spreadsheets and notes from the last two years of planning, but could be more careful in her record-keeping, putting together a more specific timeline and checklist of planning tasks. She realized that careful documentation is important, even though it can easily get overlooked.

Keeping clear documentation of the planning process is crucial because a program planner may want to look back and see where the planning process could have improved. Planners also need to look toward the future. Planning timelines or timetables can help identify and prioritize tasks for program implementation.

A **Gantt chart** organizes tasks to be completed in a series of rows. Columns represent segments of time, such as days, weeks, or months. Each task is scheduled to take a certain amount of time, depicted on the columns. As you make progress toward completing tasks, you can update the Gantt chart and affirm you are meeting deadlines as outlined. Browse Gantt chart templates available online.

SPREADING THE MESSAGE OF RECOVERY THROUGH DIFFUSION THEORY

In the future, Juli wanted to create a mission statement for the event, something that would reflect the goal of "celebration and bringing the recovery community together to support each other." **Mission statements** are designed to concisely share the purpose of the event or organization, along with an indication of who the target population is, and what activities are involved.

In Juli's case, she expressed the purpose of the event (i.e. "celebration" and "support") and indicated the target population (i.e. "recovery community") but needed to elaborate on the main activities of the Recovery Ride and Rally. It could look something like this: "The Recovery Ride and Rally aims to bring the recovery community together to celebrate and support each other through a one-day event of vendors, music, speakers, and entertainment."

She reiterated that the purpose of the Recovery Ride and Rally was to "share the positive side of recovery, which people don't always understand." She explained, "There's a lot of stigma around addiction, and a lot of times the focus is on the tragedy that we see, which can be overwhelming." With this public event, "we show our communities that there is a solution and that there's so much to be celebrated in recovery."

So, how does an idea like "We Do Recover," the motto of the Recovery Ride and Rally, spread throughout a community? How is it possible to disrupt the stigma of addiction? Effective diffusion – the process by which new ideas and practices are communicated and adopted – is the ultimate goal of an information campaign, and even benefits community members who have not directly come in contact with a program or intervention (Rogers, 2003). Diffusion theory has been used to understand how certain attitudes and practices spread throughout a community until they become widely accepted.

Diffusion theory identifies the factors that facilitate the spread of a new idea or product. The trend must be innovative enough to get people's attention, but also familiar enough that it is palatable for a common audience. In other words, if an idea is to spread, it must align to some extent with the values and practices that a community already has so that a large enough number of people can participate without feeling that there is significant risk in doing so.

It is important to identify the **early adopters**, or *opinion leaders*, because they will naturally be instrumental in proliferating health promotion programs and associated public health messages. Opinion leaders tend to be of high status, well-known, well-connected and influential within their communities. Many awareness campaigns leverage buy-in from opinion leaders to increase demand and support for services, which is especially impactful if opinion leaders put their weight behind one specific issue.

The benefit of diffusion is efficiency, as many people can be reached through just a small number of opinion leaders. With the social process of diffusion, it is possible for programs and public health messages to reach a population beyond their direct participants. Once the opinion leaders have adopted a new idea or product, the "early majority adopters" and "late majority adopters," who comprise the majority of the population (roughly 68%), decide whether a trend will hit critical mass, spread widely, and become part of the cultural fabric.

For students who want to learn more about how Diffusion Theory works in popular culture, check out Malcolm Gladwell's book *The Tipping Point.*

Diffusion typically occurs slowly, over the course of several years, so program planners need to be willing to "play the long game." This process can take even longer for interventions related to substance abuse because the social stigma often related to this condition means that people may be less likely to share information about it (Miller et al., 2006).

MEASURING THE SUCCESS OF THE EVENT THROUGH EVALUATION

How do you evaluate the impact of an event like the Recovery Ride and Rally? Juli characterized the event as a success. She noted, "We had a really good turnout and lots of participation." The rally would continue to be held each year because, as she explained, it is a relatively small investment for an activity that brings together and inspires a variety of people from the recovery community. Moreover, people "vote with their feet," meaning that they express their approval for the event by coming back to it each year.

If you want to measure the quality of the planning process, you will need to conduct a **process evaluation**. Process evaluations use timelines, checklists, and other documentation to review what to do differently the next time the event is held. It looks at what went well in planning, what went poorly, and how well program implementation followed the established plan (McKenzie et al., 2017).

If you want to measure whether people changed in some way because of the program, you will need to conduct a **summative evaluation**. Summative evaluations assess the effectiveness of the program in terms of whether awareness, attitudes, knowledge, behavior, the environment, or health status of the target population changed as a result of the program (McKenzie et al., 2017).

There was no formal process evaluation in place for the Recovery Ride and Rally event. But, informally, Juli paid attention to what was working during the event planning process and what was not, and asked others for feedback.

Based on what she observed on the day of the event, Juli said she would like to organize the layout of the venue differently. She felt that the activities were a little too spread out, and she would like to move the vendor and registration areas closer to the stage. Also, many participants seemed to miss the registration table because they were entering the event near the stage rather than across from it where the table was located. Juli said that next year she would put herself or another volunteer more regularly on the stage microphone – telling people where to go, what was going on, or what would be coming up next. She would also invite the media to cover the event. A videographer took some footage of the rally, but the event would benefit from exposure through local news channels.

Another way to assess the quality of the planning process would be to note the number of people who attended. This year, advertising materials urged attendees to preregister through an online system, provided through the Mental Health of America, called Purple Pass. Even if attendees did not donate $15 to participate in the ride or walk, they could register for free to help predict the head tally and earn some recovery swag. Juli said she would use this system again because it helped to predict attendance with some accuracy. Nearly 200 people preregistered, and she guessed correctly that over 300 would attend.

Still, the registration system was confusing for some participants who had been taking part in the event for years but had never been asked to preregister. They assumed that registration meant that they had to pay just to show up. Next year, Jodi said she would try to do a better job of letting people know that basic participation is still free. She also said she might ask participants to share demographic information (race/ethnicity, age, gender, etc.) at the time of registration to learn more about who attended the event.

In the future, a summative evaluation could be conducted, such as using a post-attendance satisfaction survey where attendees could indicate which activities they participated in and whether they felt they gained value from them. As opposed to measuring the quality of the planning process (i.e. process evaluation), impact surveys measure whether participants may have changed in some way due to the event (i.e. summative evaluation). Did they gain knowledge, skills, or resources, or experience a change in attitude? The survey could be emailed after the event to those who registered online, as well as made available to attendees on paper while at the event. This type of assessment would allow the Addiction Issues Coalition and its sponsors to know whether, and in what ways, the event met the needs of the target population. For example, a question on the survey could assess if the participant received information from any of the vendor booths and enrolled in a new service or program to maintain their sobriety as a result.

The full impact of an event like the Recovery Ride and Rally is difficult to measure with merely numbers, dollars, or surveys. Before the motorcyclists began to arrive at the start of the day, a young woman was wrapping a plastic banner, filled with photos of mostly smiling faces, around the trunk of a tree. Beneath the photos, messages written in marker and paint pen said things like, "You are forever in our hearts, forever loved, forever remembered" and "Gone but not forgotten. We love you." It was a memorial to loved ones who had been lost to alcohol and drug overdose, especially overdose due to opioids.

The sound of motorcycle engines revved in the distance. An energetic lady with short, spiky, gray hair held up a megaphone calling everyone to meet the bikers as they entered the park. A group of mostly purple and white shirts moved over in unison, past a table where children were now lining up to get their faces painted and another where they were getting purple cotton candy.

The engines were noticeably louder toward the park entrance, and motorcyclists arrived with a flourish – one-by-one or in pairs. The crowd cheered them. Then, as if on cue, the band, having tuned their instruments, began their first song.

The lady with the megaphone skipped over from where the bikers were to the area just in front of the stage and began dancing.

♪ ♫ *Don't stop…believin'…Hold on to that fee-ee-ee-lin'.* ♪ ♫

Others followed and danced along with her. A young man in a "Sober AF" t-shirt making his way to the stage area caught a passerby's eye, pointed and shouted, "Hey there!" He lifted his hand for a hi-five and met it in the air with hers. "Alright!" He skipped over to the dance area. The fellow attendee laughed with delight and followed him into the celebration.

DISCUSSION QUESTIONS

1. Why was there an emphasis on wearing specific t-shirts? What was likely the thinking behind this decision in the minds of the planners?

2. What are some benefits to incorporating corporate sponsors at public events? What would you tell a potential sponsor to try to get their support?

3. What benefits are there to having a specific fundraising goal?

4. What specific ways could a formal planning committee help Juli plan for the next Recovery Ride and Rally?

5. Who are examples you know of that represent "doers" and "influencers"? Which description fits you best, and in what situations?

6. Innovations typically begin in larger, high density, urban areas then spread out to more remote, rural areas. Can you think of a trend in which this is the case?

7. Who are examples of opinion leaders you know of? What makes them so influential? How might a planner recruit an opinion leader?

8. What might be the reasons for the main planner wanting to collect demographic data next time to see who was attending? What sort of demographic info might be useful to collect for evaluation and why? If you could only ask attendees three questions at enrollment, what would they be?

9. Does strong attendance at an event mean the event was necessarily successful? Why and why not? What was the ultimate outcome the planners of this event were hoping to accomplish? What would indicate that that outcome has been achieved?

10. How could the event organizers motivate attendees to complete a satisfaction survey?

ACTIVITIES

1. Identify all the ways the color purple was used to establish branding for recovery work.

2. Imagine you were a planning committee for this activity. Go back through the chapter and identify tasks that needed to be accomplished. Identify the type of person or agency that would be a good fit for accomplishing each task. Be sure to include a chairperson, doers, and influencers among your committee. Determine the order in which tasks would need to begin and be completed using a Gantt chart.

3. Write a mission statement for an organization that would plan this kind of activity. Keep the ultimate outcome of the activity in mind. It may help to look for definitions and models of mission statements online.

4. You are in charge of the evaluation portion of this project. Decide the process and summative outcomes you would measure to

determine the success of the activity. How would you measure them? When would you begin gathering data? How would you draw your conclusions about the success of the activity?

5. Conduct a personal assessment of your own organizational skills. How well do you maintain personal documents? Do you keep good records/notes for class or personal projects? Describe your system of personal or professional record keeping and whether you enjoy this task. Do you keep a clean and well-organized desk? Email inbox? Computer desktop? Where did you learn your habits? Have they changed over time?

REFERENCES

Clepper, R. (2023). 50 Nonprofit Fundraising Strategies to Help You Raise More. *Neon One.* https://neonone.com/resources/blog/nonprofit-fundraising-strategies/

McKenzie, J., Neiger, B., & Thackeray, R. (2017). *Planning, Implementing, and Evaluating Health Promotion Programs: A Primer* (7th ed.). USA: Pearson.

Miller, W., Sorensen, J., Selzer, J., & Brigham, G. (2006). Disseminating evidence-based practices in substance abuse treatment: A review with suggestions. *Journal of Substance Abuse Treatment, 31*(1), 25–39.

Mohebbi, B. (2014). The art of packaging: An investigation into the role of color in packaging, marketing, and branding (SSRN Scholarly Paper ID 3329815). *Social Science Research Network.* https://papers.ssrn.com/abstract=3329815

Penney, K. (2018). 3 Ways Merchandise Fundraising Attracts and Engages Donors. *Bloomerang.* https://bloomerang.co/blog/3-ways-merchandise-fundraising-attracts-and-engages-donors/

Rogers, E. (2003). *Diffusion of Innovations.* New York: Free Press of Glencoe.

CHAPTER

RED RIBBON WEEK

RAISING SUPPORT TO CHANGE COMMUNITY NORMS

In this chapter, we reflect on a drug awareness program called Red Ribbon Week. In addition to covering implementation logistics like budget development, we look through the lens of a behavioral change theory to understand how attitudes, knowledge, and behavior can be influenced through interventions.

For the past 25 years, Red Ribbon Week has been the flagship drug awareness and prevention program for the local Coordinating Council for Substance Use Prevention (CCSUP). This year, the CCSUP executive director Darby Montegro was working with an eight-person steering committee to plan and implement the Red Ribbon kick-off breakfast for guests ranging from local community members to educators, law enforcement officers, treatment providers, and social service agencies.

Health Promotion Planning: Learning from the Accounts of Public Health Practitioners,
First Edition. Jean Marie S. Place, Jonel Thaller, and Scott S. Hall.
© 2024 John Wiley & Sons, Inc. Published 2024 by John Wiley & Sons, Inc.

Many people who attended public school in the United States might remember the annual drug-free rallies and the widely distributed red ribbons with slogans embossed in gold print (e.g. "The Choice for Me is Drug Free!"). When the first Red Ribbon celebration kicked off in 1988 with a flurry of activity, every student received a stiff satin ribbon to proudly pin on their chest, the year's drug-free slogan embossed in gold print.

Red Ribbon Week began more than three decades ago, but the campaign remains the nation's largest and longest-running drug awareness and prevention program. Red Ribbon Week got its start when a Drug Enforcement Agent, Enrique "Kiki" Camarena, was brutally tortured and killed by a drug cartel. Parents and neighbors in Camarena's hometown began wearing red ribbons as a way to bring attention to the pain inflicted on their community by drug use. The ribbons were meant to signal a community-wide commitment to combat drugs.

This organization, started by parents, is still largely run by parents, and is now housed under the umbrella of the National Family Partnership and often championed by Parent Teacher Associations (PTAs) across the United States. In addition to distributing ribbons, schools are encouraged to incorporate drug prevention curriculum in classrooms for the duration of a week in late October.

Darby was new to her position at the CCSUP, replacing Sally Kingston as executive director. Sally had developed the idea for a community-wide breakfast, but as the new director, Darby focused her efforts on freshening up the planning process and dusting out excess expenses from the budget. Darby was excellent at her new job, having overseen fundraising for a public art museum for many years. This background prepared her to direct attention towards ensuring her budget would be sufficient to carry out the breakfast event.

DIVERSE SOURCES OF BUDGETARY SUPPORT

Local Coordinating Councils (LCCs) like the CCSUP are responsible for planning and coordinating the local response to drug and alcohol abuse, and often receive various sources of government funding to carry out their work. Darby had an annual budget of roughly $100,000 to work with, and she was devoting about 20% to funding the Red Ribbon Breakfast. She often thought of her budget flow like a marble run – a colorful toy her now-teenage daughters used to piece together and play with as children. Federal, state, and county funding, she said, are like marbles that are sent spinning as they drop from elevated platforms, coasting down to tracks at lower levels, and finally being deposited into buckets at the bottom. Federal funding rolls down to the state, who then announces grant opportunities to state regions. Within each region, LCCs are at the bottom of the track, vying for the whizzing marbles of available funding. She was grateful that a grant had been awarded to the CCSUP, thus parceling out federal and state funds to support the county's Red Ribbon Week.

Intergovernmental grants refer to monies transferred from the federal government to state and local governments. There are more than 200 intergovernmental grants each year in the United States that use federal money provided by taxpayers to fund state and local programs.

One disadvantage of receiving this money is that local programs may need to follow federal guidelines, which can sometimes be cumbersome. The three types of intergovernmental grants are *block grants, categorical formula grants,* and *project grants.*

Financial support from community members and local businesses are also integral to the success of Red Ribbon Week. Darby explained that she had an arsenal of funding strategies to support the Red Ribbon Breakfast, including selling $25 tickets to the breakfast to the interested public and asking community organizations to become a Red Ribbon Week sponsor. She had planned out a schedule and procedure for implementing her funding strategies. About six months prior to Red Ribbon Week, Darby drafted a "save the date" letter, announcing the upcoming breakfast and outlining different ways to financially support the event. She sent the letters to both big and small businesses, nonprofit organizations, and municipal and county-level social service agencies.

The secret, according to Darby, was to keep careful track of who had attended or donated in the past and entreat them to support the event again. The CCSUP asked organizations to consider being a sponsor for the event and providing a monetary gift, either at the Bronze level for a donation of $250, which would garner the organization a reserved table of 8 at the breakfast, acknowledgment on social media, and a mention in the event's opening PowerPoint, or a Silver-level donation of $500, where organizational names would also printed in the program. At the Gold level for $1000, an organizational logo and name would be prominently promoted at the breakfast and printed on the back of 7500 t-shirts given to the county's school children to celebrate Red Ribbon Week (the shirts sport the bubble-letter phrase "I'd Rather Eat Bugs Than Do Drugs."). The Platinum level ($1500) pulled out all the stops with wide promotion of name and logo, including on websites, Red Ribbon brochures, and on conspicuous banners that would hang on either side of the event stage.

Darby also provided a Merchant Sponsorship option that did not require a cash donation. As a merchant sponsor, for-profit businesses agreed to provide a special offer, activity, or discount to students who participated in Red Ribbon Week by wearing an emblematic Red Ribbon bracelet. The bracelets would be emblazoned with a drug-free message and distributed to all school-aged children, along with a colorful brochure highlighting various events, activities, and discounts available during the week. When the students presented their bracelet at a business, they might get two-for-one ice cream cones, a free pair of skates for the roller rink, or a 25% discount on miniature golf. As crowds patronized the business they would also be supporting a good cause.

Finally, businesses could also choose to donate products or services to be auctioned at the Red Ribbon Breakfast. Darby envisioned bright cellophaned baskets, bursting with products. She wanted the auction items to be the first thing the guests saw greeting them as they walked in the door. She joked, "I want the gleaming displays to hurt your eyes!" Products and services were previewed on social media in the weeks leading up to the breakfast, whetting attendees' appetites and priming their pocketbooks. There were baskets of lotions, incense, and spa supplies; baskets with a single gift card tipped up for the viewer; and one basket cradling a round, iced cake. Services were offered too, like family haircuts and bowling lanes with tokens for pizza. On the morning of the breakfast, attendees could indicate how much they were willing to pay to take home the prize. The CCSUP incentivized participation in the silent auction by providing businesses roughly the same benefits as a Bronze-level monetary sponsorship. Darby's hope was that the CCSUP could at least recoup $3500 from proceeds of the silent auction.

Gifts, or contributions, can be sums of money that are given voluntarily to support a program without expectation of reimbursement or compensation in return. Gifts are often referred to as *soft money* because they are offered at one point in time, as opposed to hard money which is a continuing source of funding.

Darby commented, "One thing I want to improve in future years is the sponsorship letter." She continued, "I want to tell a better story about who the CCSUP is, what Red Ribbon Week is, the reasons for holding a breakfast, and most importantly, what we will do with the money." Whether organizations decided to contribute through monetary, merchant, or silent auction sponsorship, their support was essential for keeping CCSUP programs afloat.

AWARENESS-RAISING AS A COMMUNITY-WIDE INTERVENTION

The kick-off breakfast was held on a Tuesday morning at 7 a.m. Attendees rushed from their cars in the rain and predawn darkness. One woman pulled a shawl tightly around her shoulders against the freezing rain and hurried inside the conference center. The large ballroom was teaming with people who wove in and out between 80 circular tables, each table topped with a red tablecloth, a name plate (sponsored by an organization or group of individuals from the community for a Bronze-level donation of $250), and shiny, metallic spritzes. Cascading curtains of white lights hung from the ceiling. The front stage was flanked by two banners displaying logos of local businesses sponsoring the event. The decor was like a high school Prom, though most of the breakfast attendees were closer in age to parental chaperones, all moving slowly toward an open buffet at the back of the room, hoping to get their fill of donuts and yogurt.

About 300 attendees would eventually find their way into the conference hall. Among them were representatives of nearly every community sector: the city council, educators, parents, youth, librarians, media, medical providers, helping professionals, law enforcement, business leaders, religious organizations, civic/volunteer groups, and both mayoral candidates competing in the local election, among many others. They had come to the Red Ribbon breakfast for multiple reasons, including to support the aims listed on the event flyer:

- To raise awareness of the effects of drug and alcohol abuse, especially the impact of opioids
- To celebrate and encourage positive life choices
- To remind youth and parents that drugs are present and active in neighborhoods
- To let youth know that the county cares and wants them to reach their fullest potential by living drug free

Awareness campaigns use health communication strategies to inform and influence the public.

Awareness campaigns can help change and reinforce attitudes and social norms related to health behaviors, encourage and motivate people to follow health recommendations, and increase demand for health services. They are less useful at sustaining behavior change. This may be due, in part, to the more passive role participants take when being exposed to health communication strategies. However, in some cases, people actively seek, develop, and share health information (Thackeray & Neiger, 2009).

Penetration rate is the number of people that health communication strategies reach in the target population. The penetration rate of health communication strategies is often large, given the role radio, television, websites, and social media can play in dissemination, in addition to on-on-one, small group, and organizational channels of communication.

Board member, Thomas Shinn, donning a symbolic red sweater and white turtleneck, used a microphone to welcome attendees to the 25th annual breakfast, then quickly exited to make way for the rest of the show. Forty-one teenagers rushed the event stage, members of the CCSUP youth team, performing a dance routine that included two skits: one on drunk driving and the other on vaping. Next, while breathing heavily from their dance routine, the teenagers acted as stagehands, moving a row of tables to the front of the stage to set up for a seven-person panel, as the trailer of a local documentary on the stigma of drug use played on two large screens in the background.

Panel members included a physician specializing in addiction medicine, a prosecuting attorney, a police sergeant, a health educator, a journalism professor, and the deputy state health commissioner. The teenagers roamed the crowd collecting slips of paper from audience members who had questions for the panel. The panel discussed a variety of topics – post-incarceration support, finding and prosecuting drug dealers, poverty as a social determinant of health, and medication assisted treatment. After some time, the panel began to coalesce around the need for sober living housing within the community. A local news article later recapped the panel discussion, describing it as "the start of work community leaders hoped would help provide more residential rehab programs." While bringing awareness to a need is far from implementing concrete brick-and-mortar plans, every successful community organizing effort begins with recognition of the issue.

Interventions, sometimes called *programs*, are planned actions that are designed to prevent disease or injury or promote health among a target population (McKenzie et al., 2017). A one-day event is an intervention as much as an eight-week class, a radio spot, an educational pamphlet, or a health-promoting policy change. Interventions can be made up of a single activity or multiple activities, a concept known as **multiplicity**.

Research has shown that interventions with more activities (e.g. an event, a class, a radio spot, a pamphlet, *and* a policy change) are more likely to impact the target population than interventions with a single activity. Interventions with activities on multiple levels of the socio-ecological model are especially effective, such as those that aim to address individual knowledge or beliefs, interpersonal relationships, organizational and community structures, and societal norms.

Intervention **dose** refers to the number of program units delivered. An intervention may consist of multiple activities (multiplicity) and each of those activities has an associated dose. For example, the event has one dose if it is only a one-time event. The dose of a class is eight if the class is offered once a week for eight weeks. The dose for a radio spot depends on how many radio spots would run over a period of time. The number of pamphlets distributed is the dose, along with the number of policies changed and/or developed and implemented.

Generally, the more exposure a person has to an intervention or interventions, the greater the chance for behavior change.

Most awareness campaigns alone are insufficient for inducing behavior change or reducing the risk of disease. A multi-pronged intervention to address opioid misuse, for example, should include some sort of awareness-raising, but should also likely include education and training for health professionals, expanded recovery services, universal prevention programs, medication-assisted treatment options, trauma-informed care, and poverty alleviation, among other considerations. Multi-pronged approaches are needed to move the needle on preventing and reducing complex problems like substance abuse.

The breakfast ended with the youth team performing another choreographed dance routine to a rendition of "Lean on Me." In closing remarks, the speaker announced that the youth team would bring their performance to 14 elementary schools in the county as part of drug prevention programming.

PLANNING INTERVENTIONS TO PROMOTE AND REINFORCE BEHAVIORAL CHANGE

One day after the Red Ribbon Kick-Off Breakfast, the youth team arrived at Franklin Elementary in their matching black and white t-shirts that were embellished with sponsor logos and rustling exercise pants. The troupe bounded happily into the gymnasium. A tall, blonde, young man confidently dribbled a basketball between his legs before leaping up to ceremoniously place it in the basket. The students – kindergarteners to fifth graders – gaped in awe at the effortless maneuver. Music broke out once all elementary-school students were seated and 20 youth team members transformed into one undulating, oscillating, moving mass. Their machine-like motions matched the hip-hop music, and heads popped, knees ducked, and shoulders twisted in rhythm to a Beyonce song. About three minutes into the music, a young woman burst from the group and skipped along the front row, revealing the purpose of their visit. "We are drug-free, and we are here to encourage YOU to be drug-free!" The students, enamored with the spectacle, broke out in cheers.

The dance performance was followed by skits addressing prescription pill misuse and bullying, but there were no microphones, making it almost impossible to hear the team above the wiggling and whispering of students. Team members tried occasionally to quiet the crowd by holding up their fingers bent in the form of a bird with its beak clamped shut. The final skit was a mock dance competition, pitting half of the team members dressed in black shirts against the other half in white shirts. The black-shirt dancers held red plastic cups to illustrate a party scene. They danced half-heartedly, as if drunk and dizzy, but they clearly were not a match for the white-shirt team, presumably sober, who outdid them with energetic, animated moves. The message was: Hey! Be a whiz on the dance floor, come join us, be drug free!

Although the main goal of the Red Ribbon campaign was to prevent drug use among elementary school students, it also served to prevent drug use among the youth team members. Kelsey, the team coordinator, talked about how participation on the team was beneficial to the dancers themselves, especially in the Spring when party season rolled around. "We'll sit down and talk, like, we'll sit in circles sometimes and just talk about how [parties with drugs and alcohol] affects the team. I think having those conversations with them and making sure that they feel connected to others … will reinforce them thinking like, 'Alright, I'm doing the right thing.'" Being part of the youth team reinforced abstinence from drugs and alcohol.

The *Precede-Proceed* model is a well-known health promotion planning model. Planners work to identify a desired outcome, determine what contributes to it, and design interventions to obtain it.

In the Precede-Proceed health model, it is important to understand factors that can support or hinder behavior change. They are grouped into three categories:

1. Predisposing factors include a person's knowledge, attitude, values, beliefs, and perceptions.

2. Enabling factors include access and availability to health resources and skillsets.

3. Reinforcing factors are feedback and rewards that encourage or discourage the continuation of the behavior.

What kinds of positive reinforcement can motivate behavior change? Green and Kreuter (2005), the theorists of the Precede-Proceed model, suggest that (1) social benefits, (2) physical benefits, (3) self-actualizing benefits (e.g. improving appearance, increasing self-respect, or associating with admired persons), and (4) tangible rewards (e.g. financial incentives) are salient motivators.

Members of the youth team were treated like local celebrities as they sought to reinforce positive, healthy choices. Their group image was featured on a billboard in a well-traveled part of town and full-page publicity posters were distributed in mass to school districts across the county. The **social benefits** of recognition, appreciation, and admiration helped to reinforce the team members' decisions to be sober. Over 150 students from 9 high schools had applied to be part of the team, and sometimes only 10 spots were available.

Students accepted to the team were expected to use their small-town fame to connect with other students and promote a drug-free lifestyle. This might mean spending a day eating lunch with elementary students in the school cafeteria, hanging out with younger kids at recess, or as witnessed at Franklin Elementary, reaching out to others through the dance skit and ample use of high-fives. The team members' task was to communicate the message that the social benefits of being drug-free are more desirable than those of doing drugs – and they were betting on the idea that young people wanted to hear this message from other young people. For the most part, Kelsey said the team was successful at getting drug-free behavior to be an admired behavior: "The kids look up to my students as, like actual superheroes, which is so cool because we're telling them, 'Don't do drugs, don't do alcohol,' and it's a positive impact instead of just throwing facts [at them]."

The **physical benefits** of remaining drug free were on display in every aspect of the youth team's high energy performance and their interactions with the audience. The sober group won the mock dance competition because they were sharper and more energetic than those who were drinking alcohol. Even though alcohol initially loosens inhibitions, the drug-free kids were quick on their toes and, ultimately, won the draw. The red-cup holders lost the competition, with one lamenting, "Guys, I'm having a really hard time keeping up." In the script, a peer responds, "You know, maybe they are right. We probably shouldn't be using drugs." The team members tried to communicate that remaining drug free provides you with physical benefits and drug use dulls the senses and keeps you from being your best self.

At the end of the performance, youth team members pulled trading cards out of their pockets – autographs included! – and handed them to the younger students. In one trading card, a handsome boy smiled back from a professional headshot. He would graduate high school in three years. His activities were listed on the card and included tennis, basketball, baseball, and Scouts. His drug-free message was illustrated in bubble *WordArt*: "I stay drug free so I can be my best me!" These rewards for engaging in a behavior - like improved respect and admiration - were **self-actualizing benefits** because it helped the boy feel popular and well-liked.

Kelsey described how as a young student she had collected trading cards from the generation ahead of her. It was hugely motivating to see peers glamorized on trading cards because it meant that the path to being like someone on the youth team was achievable: Just remain drug free. Five years later, she was on the team and stayed there throughout high school. She now led the team as their coordinator. She explained, "'[Team members] are trying to convey to the younger students [that] they're normal people. If there's a girl that's a second grader who's a dancer, one of my girls will go and be like, 'I'm a dancer, too. You can do it.'" Trading cards served as one way to inspire behavior change by envisioning oneself as being like the person on the card. Many kids, Kelsey said, kept the cards as bookmarks or saved them in wallets – a reminder of what they want to be.

In addition to social, physical, and self-actualizing benefits from their work on the youth team, the dancers also received tangible rewards. **Tangible rewards** included the economic benefits of engaging in a behavior. One tangible reward for seniors graduating from high school came in the form of college scholarship money. Their time spent volunteering and performing on the youth team – and success in a host of other athletic and extracurricular activities made possible through a drug-free lifestyle – was frequently rewarded by receiving a scholarship.

REVIEWING THE EVENT TO IMPROVE FUTURE PLANNING

After Red Ribbon Week was successfully implemented and done for the year, Darby and her small planning committee began the accounting process of reviewing receipts to consider what changes should be made for next year, particularly in terms of the budget. The Red Ribbon Week Breakfast was held at a fancy convention center with a 25-foot ceiling in the main ballroom and 23,400 square feet of elegantly patterned, plush carpet. It was a beautiful and convenient location, but Darby weighed the costs of using the space for next year's Red Ribbon Breakfast. Despite its "glass-enclosed pavilion, outdoor terrace, and classical splendor," as stated in the promotional materials, Darby was cognizant of the accompanying costs. On a $20,000 budget, it was tough to spend $8 on a pot of coffee or $32 per dozen donuts, especially when she could go to a local bakery and pick up the same box for $11. The curtains of light cost $900 in total, and it would have cost $27 to put out a flag (Darby opted to have a digital flag waving on the large screens, alternating between displays of sponsors' business logos). The convention center bundled food, space, and services together. The in-house catering service had to be used, along with the onsite audiovisual office, making the overall experience convenient but pricey. In Darby's case, the bundling of services made it so that she was unable to shop around for other less expensive options.

Various resources are needed to carry out program planning, many of which cost money. General categories of resources include personnel, curriculum or instructional resources, space, equipment, and supplies.

It is important to consider the financial objectives of the program – whether to turn a profit, break even, or spend money. **Accounting** consists of analyzing incoming funds and outgoing expenditures and considering the effect of these transactions on the program budget.

A **budget** is a document that lists estimated **revenues**, or sources of financial support, with **expenditures**, or costs, associated with a program. When designing a budget, consider the financial objective of the program – is it to make money? If so, how much (i.e. profit margin)? To secure a profit, expenditures should be less than the revenue.

Program budgets should be comprised of multiple sources of financial support, including in-kind contributions, participant fees, event sponsorship, third-party support, or grant funding (see Chapter 4 for more detail).

Effective budgeting requires attention to detail. Expenditures should be **itemized**, which means that each cost should be clearly listed and explained.

Two main categories of costs need to be considered in a budget:

- **Direct costs** are expended in providing services or program. They include wages, salaries, and supplies for program planning, implementation, or evaluation.
- **Indirect costs** are expended indirectly and cover overhead or administrative costs not directly associated with a program, such as electricity, utilities, insurance, and maintenance.

Darby brought up her concerns about the cost of the convention center during the following month's Board of Directors meeting. What other facilities could host the breakfast in the future to lower the costs? If a cheaper yet suitable location could be found, more of the raised funds could be retained to help supplement the CCSUP's other programs. Considering record-breaking ticket sales the previous year, the discussion centered around what local facility could hold over 700 people. There was the community art center or the community college, but their maximum capacity was capped at 450. After exploring additional options, Darby sent an email to propose the County Fairgrounds. The metal frame building with aluminum siding usually housed 4-H shows – a drawback at first glance – but held up to 775 people with a cost of only $600. The planning committee quickly responded with votes of support. The program coordinator for the local Tobacco Free Coalition responded with an important consideration: "I know their building is tobacco-free as that is our county law, but were you able to open discussion about their grounds policy? … I would like our location to be in support of our [drug-free] message." No one responded to his message, perhaps indicating that logistical concerns – like capacity and cost – sometimes outweigh the desire to align practice with policy.

Because the space rental at the county fairgrounds was not bundled with food services, the planning committee was planning to hire an external vendor to provide food for attendees for next year's breakfast. For the next year, Darby wanted to move away from a warm breakfast of pancakes and sausages to platters of pre-prepared breakfast items. This move would save almost $7000 dollars, but some long-time board members worried about the quality declining. Darby's response was concise: "If you're here for the food, you're here for the wrong reason." This was her way of ensuring that planning stayed focused on achieving the program's goals. "It is always such a balance, trying to manage the budget and other logistics, but trying to keep all of us focused on the overall goal: promoting a drug-free community," noted Darby.

DISCUSSION QUESTIONS

1. What are the benefits of increasing public awareness of an issue as part of a prevention program?

2. Can you think of any downsides to focusing on wearing ribbons to promote a message? Explain.

3. What might be some specific challenges of implementation in programs that target children? What extra factors might need to be accounted for when planning for such programs?

4. The claim was made that young people like to hear messages presented to them by other young people. Why might that be? What precautions might you take when using young people to deliver a message?

5. Would the youth team's message resonate with a middle or high school crowd? Why or why not?

6. The chapter talks about reinforcing factors for behavior change. What are some predisposing and enabling factors that would support substance use prevention?

7. If you were to take over a program that has a long history of doing things a certain way, and you believed some of those things needed to change, how can you go about implementing those changes without losing the support from stakeholders?

8. Based on the four aims of the Red Ribbon campaign described in the flyer for the kickoff breakfast, and the descriptions provided in the chapter of the program, how well do you think each of those aims were addressed by the efforts of those facilitating the program? Explain.

9. What public awareness campaigns do you remember seeing or participating in? How effective do you think they were?

10. Is raising awareness enough? The US has almost 200 official health awareness days, but there is little evidence that awareness campaigns actually incite change. Is there a better way to bring change to issues like the opioid crisis?

11. How should a planner balance the preferences of stakeholders with the realities of a budget?

12. How would you go about setting sponsorship levels for local businesses?

ACTIVITIES

1. Imagine you are tasked with creating a slogan for a public awareness campaign for high school students related to one of the following: encouraging dental hygiene, discouraging vaping, discouraging cyber-bullying, encouraging in-person activities instead of screen time, or other. Come up with a slogan and some kind of public signal students can use (e.g. the red ribbon) that you think would be motivating for adolescents. Explain your reasoning.

2. Investigate a public awareness campaign that you find online. Evaluate the following:

   - What was done to make the issue more visible (increase public awareness)?

   - How clear are the objectives of the campaign?

   - What gives you confidence that the campaign would be successful?

   - What makes you doubtful that the campaign would be successful?

   - How would you improve the campaign?

3. Imagine you are preparing to approach a sponsor to ask for donations that will help increase public awareness among high school students of one of the following topics: encouraging dental hygiene, discouraging vaping, discouraging cyber-bullying, encouraging in-person activities instead of screen time, or other. Based on the *Precede-Proceed* model, help motivate the potential sponsor to see the potential community impact of sponsorship by describing at least three benefits of behavior change for each of the following categories: (1) social benefits, (2) physical benefits, (3) self-actualizing benefits, and (4) tangible rewards.

REFERENCES

Green, L. & Kreuter, M. (2005). *Health Program Planning: An Educational and Ecological Approach* (4th ed.). Boston, MA: McGraw-Hill.

McKenzie, J., Neiger, B., & Thackeray, R. (2017). *Planning, Implementing, and Evaluating Health Promotion Programs: A Primer* (7th ed.). USA: Pearson.

Thackeray, R. & Neiger, B. (2009). A multidirectional communication model: Implications for social marketing practice. *Health Promotion Practice, 10*, 2, 171–175.

CHAPTER

THE WISE PROGRAM

SOCIAL MARKETING STRATEGIES TO PROMOTE HEALTH EDUCATION INTERVENTIONS

In this chapter, we highlight a program coordinator discussing social marketing strategies to expand the number of participants in the WISE program – a health education curriculum for seniors that incorporates some substance use content. As the program expands its reach, she also discusses the important role of setting up proper formative and summative evaluations.

The office for the local Coordinating Council for Substance Use Prevention (CCSUP) is located amid a cluster of small businesses, specialized medical offices, and a large, tent-like batting cage. Darby Montegro, the Executive Director, had called a special meeting to discuss a recruitment challenge. A program under her watch was struggling to deliver its content to enough people. She needed to reach at least 50 individuals to satisfy the stipulations of the grant her office had received.

Health Promotion Planning: Learning from the Accounts of Public Health Practitioners,
First Edition. Jean Marie S. Place, Jonel Thaller, and Scott S. Hall.
© 2024 John Wiley & Sons, Inc. Published 2024 by John Wiley & Sons, Inc.

The program is called the Wellness Initiative for Senior Education (WISE), which is an evidence-based program to promote healthy lifestyle choices and prevent substance misuse among adults ages 55 and older (New Jersey Prevention Network [NJPN], 2008). Focusing a program on a homogenous segment of society (i.e. segmentation; see more information in Chapter 3) can help target information to fit a clear set of needs, but, in this case, narrowing a program to a specific age group made it more difficult to find enough interested people to participate.

WISE was created by the New Jersey Prevention Network (NJPN) and launched in 1996. It has spread throughout the United States to serve over 40,000 people.

The curriculum consists of six weekly sessions that last two to three hours and typically includes breakfast or lunch. Sessions include a variety of delivery modes such as lecture, discussion, small group activities, and individual exercises. Tools and resources for use at home are also provided to help reinforce what participants learn. Participants are encouraged to share information with others (Administration for Community Living [ACL], 2011).

THE BENEFITS OF USING A CANNED PROGRAM FOR HEALTH EDUCATION

At the CCSUP, three retirement-aged WISE program facilitators and a staff member from a local nonprofit joined Darby in the office conference room. Darby explained the situation to the team of women, hoping to generate new recruiting avenues for potential program participants. Immediately, Fanny, a trained WISE facilitator, declared that the classes she teaches are "active and fun" but worried that people probably assume they are too formal. Heads nodded in unison while others verbally confirmed the claim. They assured themselves: If they could just help the **target population** – those whom they hope will participate in the program – see how much fun the workshops are, people would be coming in droves.

Health education interventions are planned learning experiences, such as classes, courses, seminars, or workshops, that provide knowledge and skills and that happen in a formal educational setting (McKenzie et al., 2017).

Researchers Minelli and Breckon (2009) have distilled learning principles that are useful to planners who implement health education programs:

1. Incorporate learners' senses, such as seeing, hearing, and speaking
2. Design activities so learners are actively involved rather than a passive recipient
3. Eliminate distractions as much as possible in the learning environment
4. Encourage the learner to come to the program ready to participate
5. Ensure that the content has personal relevance to the learner
6. Use repetition in building learners' understanding of concepts
7. Recognize and encourage the learner in his/her process of learning
8. Strategically introduce concepts from simple and known to complex and unknown
9. Demonstrate how concepts are generalizable to other settings and situations
10. Pace lessons and material appropriately

Fanny was an older woman with a buoyant personality packed into a 5-foot frame. Working with other seniors energized her. She generally attended meetings in a royal blue jogging suit and sneakers, so full of energy that she clapped people on the back, kissed women and men on the cheek, and interjected into every conversation. Fanny commented, "I love the interactive approach in the WISE program. It's so fun for me to help these folks see what there is to celebrate in their lives, and the things they should be avoiding."

Fanny had become a trained facilitator of the WISE program by attending a two-day, off-site training, for a cost of $425 plus roundtrip travel. She had facilitated more than a dozen classes for seniors in her community in the past few years, and she had learned through experience how to reach adult learners. Based on the research Bryan et al. (2009) conducted on adult learning, she always tried to elaborate on why the material was important to the participants. For example, she discussed that everyone has idle prescription medication above their kitchen sink, and it was critical to know what to do with the unused pills. She talked about building on participants' knowledge and respecting their diverse experiences and backgrounds. "The one thing people don't want when they come to a program is to be talked down to!" she emphasized. The WISE program uses problem solving and small group discussion in each session because these approaches have been shown to be effective among adult learners.

As a trained facilitator of the WISE program, Fanny had been provided a facilitator's guide, implementation binder, and other loose leaf copies of curricular activities she could use to photocopy and give to participants. Fanny laughed at herself as she described how often she had read through her facilitator's guide, second only to her familiarity with the Bible. This guide, sometimes called a training manual or a program procedural manual, was useful because it provided a generalized guide a trained facilitator could use to run the program. She appreciated it because it structured how she approached each session, giving her ideas for discussion and providing background information on certain topics. Fanny said, "Having the additional background information on things like metabolisms and bad reactions to drugs, and so forth, it was really helpful. I didn't want to stumble over my thoughts when I'm in front of the group," she laughed again and patted the facilitator's guide in front of her. True to her word, she had brought it to this meeting. "It's been a real faithful little friend," she said.

Program procedural manuals are essential to help standardize programs. They ensure that anyone who is associated with a program understands how to implement it, thus making the program replicable in more than one setting.

Program fidelity means programs have been implemented properly, according to a preestablished plan. Program procedural manuals help ensure program facilitators implement the right content in the appropriate format as planned.

The CCSUP used funds to purchase the WISE curriculum from the New Jersey Prevention Network (NJPN). The fact that it was priced reasonably at $100 was good news given that other for-profit vendors sell curriculum for thousands of dollars, which would have limited the CCSUP's ability to purchase a canned program. At the same time, if Darby would have had to create **a program in-house**, meaning developing custom-made instructional materials, it also would have cost her extensive time, money, and effort – something that the CCSUP lacked as Darby was currently the only full-time employee on staff.

The canned program offered by NJPN was aimed at a general population 55 and over, which fit the county's target population composed of middle income folks who racially identified as Black or White. Custom-made instructional materials would have been useful if they needed to be culturally-tailored for a target population that contained specific cultural characteristics.

A **canned program**, or a program developed by an outside vendor, includes materials necessary to implement a program, such as participant's manual, instructor's manual, audiovisual materials, training materials, and marketing materials.

The WISE program materials were reviewed by an outside evaluator for overall quality and provided a score, from 0 to 4, based on three categories: implementation materials (score 2.8), training and support (score 2.5), and quality assurance (score 2.5), making its overall score a 2.6.

Program strengths included:

- Step-by-step guidance for implementation
- Materials are well-organized and easy to use
- Training includes discussion on participant recruitment
- Implementation checklists, participation evaluation forms, process data collection tools, and participant surveys are provided to support quality assurance

Weaknesses included:

- Lack of information on facilitator qualifications
- Lack of guidance on how to address the heterogeneity of the older adult population
- Unclear guidance on how interested individuals would sign up for training to be a program facilitator
- Lack of information on technical support for program implementation

Another way to evaluate the appropriateness of curriculum and other instructional materials is to use a SAM Scoring Sheet, which is a *Suitability Assessment of Materials* (SAM) instrument (Doak et al., 1996).

The WISE program has a six-lesson curriculum, each of which is taught once a week. The lessons cover changes associated with aging, cultural and generational diversity, and quality of life. In the fourth and fifth week, participants cover topics related to substance misuse, specifically medication misuse and addiction. A selection of the program goals focused on substance use includes helping seniors:

- Increase knowledge on the prevalence of medication use and factors that lead to misuse among seniors
- Ask relevant questions to healthcare providers on medication use
- Consider how medications metabolize

- Understand addiction as a disease
- Identify the signs of alcohol abuse
- Become familiar with treatment options for addiction

Health education programs provide the opportunity for participants to gain in-depth knowledge on a subject or range of related subjects.

Health education programs typically use **curriculum**, or a planned set of lessons designed to provide knowledge and competence in an area.

A curriculum's **scope** refers to the range of material covered in a program (breadth), as well as how much information is discussed within each topical area (depth).

A curriculum's sequence refers to the order in which material is presented (i.e. from simple to complex, or starting at one topic and moving to another topic) (McKenzie et al., 2017).

USING THE FOUR P'S OF SOCIAL MARKETING TO DO FORMATIVE RESEARCH

Darby, Fanny, and others at the table wondered aloud what it would take to get people interested in the WISE program. Could they make the program something that seniors get excited about? Their social marketing efforts needed to clearly tap into the wants and needs of the targeted individuals to generate interest and increase program attendance. Darby reflected on what older adults might value. Was it grandkids? Independence? Pending vacations or their pension fund? Darby and Fanny thought about how to leverage the target population's values in recruitment efforts. They were interested in taking a consumer-based planning approach that used principles of marketing to make it desirable for participants to engage in the program.

Social marketing refers to designing programs to facilitate voluntary behavior changes that result in improved well-being (Andreasen, 1995). The four "Ps" of social marketing, also known as the *marketing mix*, include product, price, place, and promotion.

Product refers to the service program planners are offering. It should meet the needs of the target population in an easy and convenient way and provide a benefit that they value.

Price refers to what it might cost the target population in time, money, or effort to obtain the product and the promised benefits.

Place refers to where the target population can access the product.

Promotion is the communication strategy used to let the target population know about the product, where and how to access it, and its associated benefits.

In a marketing sense, the WISE program was the product, and the physical, emotional, or financial efforts involved with participating were the price. The community room of a local assisted living center was the place where the WISE program was currently held. Darby had various promotion strategies to inform the public about the classes, mostly through email blasts to service providers who work with an older adult population, as well as flyers posted around town and word of mouth.

The group looked at hard copies of the promotional flyer on the table in front of them. They had distributed the flyer to churches and other places of worship, and they posted it to bulletin boards in grocery boards and mailed it to residents in assisted living. The placement of the flyer was aimed to market the program to the target population. It contained the following headline: "Are you 60 or older and looking for an opportunity to learn how to stay healthy and meet new people?" Free refreshments and giveaways were highlighted as additional benefits. Darby reminded the group that the CCSUP has a storage closet full of potential giveaways for participants – ice packs, medicine organizers, pens – that could be thrown in to sweeten the deal, if needed.

Darby asked the group if they thought the refreshments and giveaways sounded enticing enough. Participants who completed the program would also receive a gift card, but Darby expressed some reluctance about adding that information to the advertisement, wondering if it would be perceived as "tacky." She feared people might focus too much on the monetary reward instead of the educational and social benefits of attending the program.

An **incentive** is a reward for participating in a program or changing a behavior. Incentives often include money, food, or a form of special recognition. Haveman (2010) offered six guidelines for using incentives that can motivate program participation:

- Identify the desired outcome (what the program is supposed to achieve)

- Identify the behavior change (what program participants should do differently)
- Determine effectiveness of the incentive to promote the behavior change (will it work?)
- Link the incentive to the desired outcome or behavior (it directly rewards the change)
- Identify possible adverse effects of the incentive (avoid causing any harm)
- Evaluate and report behavior changes or outcomes in response to incentives (did the incentives work and how can you share what you learned about incentives)

If a program is grant funded, it is important to consider what the parameters are regarding how the funding can be used, including the purchasing of food or providing refreshments as an incentive.

Some grants do not allow for the funding to be directly allocated toward purchasing food, but some pay general stipends to an organization (as compensation for their time and efforts) that could then be used at the organization's discretion to buy refreshments.

To be eligible for future funding, it is critical to strictly follow the funder's rules.

Incentives help reduce, or compensate for, the price of participation (Haveman, 2010). For an individual who has chronic pain or social anxiety, coming to a community-based program may be a steep, effort-laden price to pay. Receiving a gift card, on the other hand, could offset some of those efforts. But maybe, Fanny suggested, they were advertising the wrong benefits. Could it be that seniors would be more driven to attend if they knew social relationships are strengthened through the program? A brief discussion ensued about how isolated people are, sticking within their own shrinking social circles. Maybe seniors simply want more friends, which would be a benefit that could drive behavior change.

Moving on, the group spent a few minutes brainstorming ways to get the word out to more people. Maybe, Fanny considered, churches could start hosting the WISE sessions in their buildings, or housing complexes that attract seniors could serve as hosts. What about targeting subsidized housing complexes, social clubs, and libraries? Choosing a place where people have easy access to the product could help ensure participation – as noted in the marketing matrix. Fanny emphasized this point. She asked again, "Was the program truly easy for someone to attend?" For an individual who does not like to drive – or cannot drive at all – providing a vehicle to pick up participants could also ease the burden substantially. Another gray-haired woman at the table suggested offering the program in the evenings for those who were not yet retired. Fanny and Darby welcomed this suggestion because it showed sensitivity to sub-groups within the target population.

Additional strategies were discussed for informing more people about the program. Someone mentioned mass emailing individuals who had previously attended a WISE session to encourage them to recruit friends, neighbors, and family members to participate in the program. Darby mentioned adding information about the WISE program to a virtual newsletter that was sent to those who participated in other programs offered by the CCSUP. These forms of promotion, along with the flyer mentioned above, would communicate messages about the nature and importance of the program, hoping to convince the target population of the benefits that come from participating in the program.

When promoting a program, McDonald and Wilson (2011) recommend keeping in mind the four purposes of communication marketing. Promotion should achieve the following:

- Inform the public about a service
- Persuade people to get involved
- Reinforce awareness of the program
- Differentiate or explain how the program is different from others

In promotional materials, it is also important to include the benefits of participation in the program, as well as information on how the public can access the program.

After a lull, someone reminded the rest of the group that the WISE classes "are really fun" and that participants "come alive." The facilitators shared anecdotes from their classes and smiles and warm laughter followed. One facilitator reported that she always held graduation ceremonies with makeshift hats and gowns. Some of the older adults had never participated in a graduation ceremony and appreciated this opportunity. Darby noted that such a ceremony could also serve as an incentive for participation. Trophies and knickknacks from the dollar store also seemed to bring joy to the participants. This was fortunate, Darby noted, because the socioeconomic circumstances of program participants are typically relevant to the types of reward deemed motivating, with wealthier populations needing higher financial rewards to feel enticed (Haveman, 2010).

Finally, Darby made an executive decision. For now, instead of consolidating class sessions, she would take the approach of over-scheduling the sessions to reach as many people as possible, which would result in small group sizes but plenty of times to choose from. She would also engage in continuous monitoring to assess the program's functioning – a type of formative evaluation – by reaching out to current participants and getting their feedback on the program. What insights could participants potentially share about how to improve the program? What should change in the program recruitment strategies? What could she learn about barriers to participation? This very meeting where they were discussing their marketing approach with her program facilitators could also be considered formative research, and she would continue her formative research until the program was the best that it could be.

Formative research or evaluation seeks to improve a program by considering changes in program components that can be integrated pre-implementation or mid-implementation.

Questions to consider in formative research include:

- Is the program justified by needs assessment data?
- Is the program evidence-based? (i.e. the program has documented data that supports its effectiveness)
- Do the professionals involved have adequate knowledge and skills to implement the program? Are there a range of professionals from different sectors involved?
- Are there adequate resources to implement the program?
- Is the program oriented to the target population based on consumer preferences?
- Are there multiple activities built into the program that address different levels of the socio-ecological model (i.e. **multiplicity**)?
- Is support for behavior change built into the program?
- Are there mechanisms built in to adapt the program based on feedback?
- Are recruitment strategies adequate and culturally appropriate?
- Is the target population provided adequate opportunity to participate in the program?
- Are professionals interacting with the target population appropriately?
- Are the needs of the target population being met through the program?

PLANNING FOR A SUMMATIVE PROGRAM EVALUATION IN THE FUTURE

After formative research, the team would ultimately need to consider an evaluation process where they could measure the impact of the hopefully new and improved program on the participants themselves. Even though the group was still in the process of doing formative research, they also needed to consider a summative evaluation.

The term **summative evaluation** is an umbrella term for evaluations that measure intermediate and long-term impacts of the program on participants.

An *impact evaluation* focuses on intermediate changes, such as participants' awareness, knowledge, attitudes, skills, behavior, and environment.

An *outcome evaluation* uses vital statistics and trend data to focus on the program's long-term effects in a population, such as mortality, morbidity, disability, the **prevalence** of something (e.g. total number of cases of a disease), or the **incidence** of something (e.g. new cases of a disease). To conduct an outcome evaluation, one must be aware of confounding variables, which are influences outside of the program that may have an impact on results.

If the group waited too long to set up summative evaluation procedures, conducting a meaningful evaluation would become increasingly difficult. Evaluations that are set up effectively from the beginning can rely on more rigorous methods that produce more informative results. For example, gathering data from participants before they begin the WISE program would be essential for measuring changes in knowledge, attitudes, and behaviors that correspond with participation in the program. A **pretest/posttest** model would allow evaluators to compare what people knew or how they acted before the program intervention with their knowledge and behavior after the intervention. Fanny laughed at the thought of not doing a pretest. "If you don't do a pretest on the first day of the program, you reach the end of the program and you're going to have to ask people what they thought they knew and acted like before they learned so much. They won't be able to tell you a thing because they won't be able to remember!" Relying on the memories and perceptions of program participants to assess how much they think they have changed is problematic because of **recall bias**, or the tendency to remember the past incorrectly. Such **retrospective** research is less reliable.

Darby was confident that the WISE program would have a positive intermediate and long-term effect. She anticipated that knowledge and behaviors of program participants would change, and that outcome indicators like morbidity and mortality would improve as well. She had investigated the WISE program before purchasing the curriculum and knew the program was highly evidence-based due to the results of multiple summative evaluations.

The New Jersey Prevention Network (NJPN) worked with the Institute for Families in the Rutgers School of Social work to conduct an impact evaluation on the program. The evaluation team identified indicators of program success, determined how to gather data, and decided how to measure the outcomes.

One major indicator they evaluated was knowledge of attitudes about alcohol and medications, aging, and depression. Participants from six New Jersey counties were randomly assigned to either participate in the six-week WISE program or do nothing different (those from this second group were able to do the program once the evaluation was completed). All participants completed a pretest survey about their knowledge of topics related to the effects of alcohol on the mind and body and on early signs of depression, along with their attitudes about aging. They completed the same survey after 6 weeks and then again after another 30 days.

Results showed that those who went through the program increased in knowledge about alcohol and aging, had improved well-being, and gained more positive attitudes toward aging, whereas no substantial changes occurred for the group who skipped the program.

Darby was interested in replicating the NJPN study among her own group of participants – if she could find enough of them! She could potentially learn more about how well the program addressed the distinctive needs of her community. In addition, based on formative research, she could adjust the program implementation in the future. As a detail-oriented person, she loved the idea of doing robust evaluation studies for the myriad of programs the CCSUP administered across the county. Part of her job was filtering through potential program curriculums located on the *Evidence-Based Practices Resource Center*. She was drawn to programs with a strong evidence base, especially those that established a comparison or control group in summative evaluation studies. She had been in the field long enough to understand that sometimes people change or improve over time regardless of whether they participate in a certain program – a type of confounding variable.

But, having a control group can help establish the validity of the evaluation results. Darby, a self-proclaimed "data nerd," enjoyed talking about the importance of using experimental designs in the evaluation of the CCSUP's programs.

An **experimental design** seeks to manipulate a variable to determine whether the variable causes a certain outcome. In the case of program evaluation, taking the program versus not taking the program is the manipulated variable. The average outcomes of a treatment and a control group are then compared.

A **control group** is comprised of similar people to those in a treatment group (those who were in the program), but do not receive the intervention or program.

A **confounding variable** is an influence that obscures the cause-and-effect relationship between variables. It could contribute to changes regardless of whether someone is part of the treatment or control group. For example, people generally feel less depressed as the seasons change from winter to spring. If the control group was evaluated during the winter and the treatment group evaluated during spring, any improvements present in the treatment group but not in the control group would be suspect. Both groups should be evaluated during the same time span (and conducted in the same way) to account for possible confounding variables.

If people are **randomly assigned** to the treatment group and the control group, and they take the same pretests at the same time, and then the same posttests at the same time, and the only major difference between the groups is participation in the program, one can have more confidence that any changes in the treatment group that do not appear in the control group are because of the intervention. In random assignment to either the control or the treatment group, everyone has an equal chance of being assigned to either group.

The *Evidence-Based Practices Resource Center* (formerly known as the *National Registry of Evidence-based Programs and Practices*) is hosted by the Substance Abuse and Mental Health Services Administration (SAMHSA). The Resource Center houses a collection of scientifically-based resources for various audiences, including ratings of programs based on the extent to which they are based on scientific evidence (see https://www.samhsa.gov/resource-search/ebp).

Darby sighed. There was so much work to be done to implement the WISE program among the target population and to evaluate it properly. She would love to have the means to hire a team of external evaluators to help her invest in an experimental design with random assignment to groups, but she also acknowledged the limitations of her organization. She was a one-woman staff with an enthusiastic, but small, group of volunteer retirees. She had a vision for what could be accomplished but moved forward one plodding step at a time. Using a canned, evidence-based program gave her some reassurance that the work they would do had a good chance of making a difference in the community.

DISCUSSION QUESTIONS

1. What do you think is the most appropriate way to advertise the program? Should the group highlight the value of the program or focus on promoting the financial rewards for participation? Which is more persuasive? What does the need for incentives say about human nature?

2. What will motivate the seniors in this group? What will make it easier for them to participate? How can you find this out?

3. How do you get the word out in an age in which people are bombarded with invitations to participate in various services and with so many scams?

4. What are the different kinds of "costs" involved with participating in a program besides money?

5. Why would having pre- and post-data be more reliable than having participants retrospectively report their attitudes, beliefs, or behaviors?

6. What might make it difficult to set up a reliable experimental evaluation of a program?

ACTIVITIES

1. Imagine you were to deliver a parallel program to the WISE program but for middle school children and their parents, focusing on the risks of drug use and signs of drug use risks (e.g. depression). Address the product, price, plan, and promotion elements of delivering this program. Create a marketing plan that follows the six bullets regarding the use of incentives. Make decisions that you think will lead to the highest participation of this target population.

2. For the scenario above, develop an evaluation of the program using the concepts described in the chapter. Come up with what you believe would be the most trustworthy evaluation. Be sure to determine the impacts and outcomes you hope to achieve and measure, how you will measure those impacts and outcomes, and when and how you would gather data. Be prepared to defend your decisions.

REFERENCES

Administration for Community Living (ACL) (2011). Wellness Initiative for Senior Education (WISE) https://acl.gov/sites/default/files/programs/2017-03/WISE_ACL_Summary.pdf

Andreasen, A. (1995). *Marketing Social Change. Changing Behavior to Promote Health, Social Development, and the Environment.* San Francisco: Jossey-Bass.

Bryan, R., Kreuter, M., & Brownson, R. (2009). Integrating adult learning principles into training for public health practice. *Health Promotion Practice, 10*(4), 557–563.

Doak, C., Doak, L., & Root, J. (1996). *Teaching Patients with Low Literacy Skills* (2nd ed.). Philadelphia, PA: J.b. Lippincott.

Haveman, R. (2010). Principles to guide the development of population health incentives. *Preventing chronic disease, 7*(5), 1–5.

McDonald, M. & Wilson, H. (2011). *Marketing Plans* (7th ed.). United Kingdom: Wiley.

McKenzie, J., Neiger, B., & Thackeray, R. (2017). *Planning, Implementing, and Evaluating Health Promotion Programs: A Primer* (7th ed.). Pearson.

Minelli, M. & Breckon, D. (2009). *Community Health Education: Settings, Roles, and Skills* (5th ed.). Sudbury, MA: Jones & Bartlett.

New Jersey Prevention Network (2008). *Wellness Initiative for Senior Education Curriculum and Training Manual.* Lakewood, NJ: Author.

New Jersey Prevention Network (2008), Wellness Initiative for Senior Education (WISE) and Wellness Initiative for Senior Education (WISE) Program: Key Evaluation Findings. https://www.njpn.org/_files/ugd/fbbd59_b1f884c0d5a547c9aad69486f57aced3.pdf

CHAPTER

7

PEER-RUN WARMLINE

MANAGING AND EVALUATING A HEALTH COMMUNICATION PROGRAM

In this chapter, we share an account of an executive director running a peer-based nonprofit. She uses health coaching and social learning to support behavioral change through modeling and reinforcement. Her experiences with staffing, training, and logic models can provide insight into health promotion organizations who do the work of program planning.

Nikki Farmston, a studious-looking woman who stands nearly 6 ft tall and proudly announces over a decade of sobriety, lives and breathes peer education. She explained, "Change is easier when other people are supportive and also behaving in similar ways."

Nikki took this truth with her as she began volunteering for Consumer Help, a peer-run, nonprofit organization in operation since

Health Promotion Planning: Learning from the Accounts of Public Health Practitioners, First Edition. Jean Marie S. Place, Jonel Thaller, and Scott S. Hall.

1992. At Consumer Help, peer support is offered to callers through the warmline, providing understanding, validation, and day-to-day practical guidance to people who cannot reach help in a clinical setting. **Peer-support**, in this case, refers to the fact that individuals who are struggling with substance use can speak over the phone with a person who has had similar struggles. Nikki started off as a warmline operator, wanting to give back to a recovery movement that saved her life from a substance use disorder. Gradually, she added office manager to her list of volunteer duties. Then, 10 years later, she was hired as the agency's executive director. The board of directors posted a job opening, did a search, and she recalled with modesty and humor, "I guess they decided I was the right fit."

The **executive director (ED)** of a nonprofit organization is similar to the chief executive officer (CEO) of a corporation. Both are responsible for administration of tasks related to daily operations and strategic planning, and must report to a board of directors.

A **board of directors** is a group of stakeholders, appointed or elected, who supervise an organization or corporation.

In her description of current programming, Nikki noted that Consumer Help facilitates skill-building workshops and support groups but is best known for their peer-run warmline, which is funded by a yearly grant from the state's Division of Mental Health and Addictions (DMHA).

A warmline supplements, but does not replace, traditional mental health and substance use services. But for callers who may be physically isolated and lack easy access to services, like those who live in rural counties, a warmline is a lifeline. Nikki noted that warmlines are particularly important for addiction, which is an incredibly lonely disease. The anonymity of telephone communication can often facilitate difficult disclosure by those who might be embarrassed or feel ashamed of their circumstances.

Hotline operators are available to respond to people in crisis 24 hours a day and 7 days a week. In a crisis, callers have immediate physical or emotional needs that overcome their current resources or coping strategies. They may be at risk of harming themselves or others.

Most hotlines include access to Spanish-speaking operators and online chat options, as well as TTY tech for people with deafness. Some mental health hotlines include:

- The National Suicide Prevention Lifeline 1-800-273-TALK or dial 988
- The National Domestic Violence Hotline 1-800-799-7233
- SAMHSA National Mental Health Helpline 1-800-662-HELP

Warmline services differ from hotlines because they are not intended for immediate crisis intervention. Rather, the person who answers a warmline, often referred to as the warmline operator, attempts to intervene *before* a situation reaches crisis status. Some warmlines operate 24/7, like hotlines, but most have limited hours and cater to a certain region or state.

BEHAVIORAL CHANGE CONCEPTS UNDERPIN WARMLINE IMPLEMENTATION

Every Monday through Friday from 8 a.m. to 4 p.m., callers struggling with addiction and other mental health issues can contact Consumer Help's peer-run warmline to speak with an operator who knows about recovery and empowerment. Nikki noted that some callers are so physically or emotionally isolated that they may not speak with anyone all day except for the operator who answers the line. Many callers are repeat callers, which can be typical for warmlines in general.

Each exchange begins with a warmline operator asking a series of questions to determine what the caller might need. The operator can offer social support in several forms, each meeting callers' different needs. At Consumer Help, an operator may provide a caller with ideas, suggestions, or referrals.

Warmline operators may offer callers a combination of **support**:

- *Emotional support* is helping a person to express feelings about things that are important to them.
- *Instrumental support* is helping a person obtain items or services of benefit to them.
- *Informational support* is helping a person gain knowledge and understanding of relevant subjects or processes.
- *Appraisal support* is helping a person by providing them with analysis and feedback that facilitates their growth.

Warmline callers request information about a variety of services and topics. Some are related directly to mental health and addiction; others are more tangential, though no less important, such as transportation, employment, and safety services. Often callers request support in navigating toxic relationships with friends or family members.

Operators can provide generic information or advice if the caller requests, but often they will simply listen and reflect what they are hearing back to the caller, providing emotional support and guiding them to identify their own solutions. The operator always tries to remind the caller that someone cares and has been through similar circumstances. Nikki asserted that the main goal of warmline services is to remind callers of "their resiliency and strength and that they have a lot of power in how they can respond to whatever is going on in their life." A conversation may unfold like this:

WARMLINE
CALLER: *"I've never felt so alone. I'm a horrible person.*
                 The pills are my only real friends."

WARMLINE
OPERATOR: *"You're not a bad person–you're NOT your addiction.*
                 I know because I used to be where you are. My life
                 is so much better now, and I want you to know that
                 you're not alone and there's hope."

Warmline operators can be considered a type of **health coach** who assists callers identify goals and uses behavioral psychological principles to help them reach goals.

Part of peer health education through warmline contact is the opportunity for **social learning,** also known as social cognitive theory (Rotter, 1954; Bandura, 1977; Bandura, 1986). The following concepts are relevant to behavior change in a warmline encounter:

- *Positive reinforcement* can be direct if someone provides verbal praise or a reward to another person, or vicarious if a person is observing another person receive praise or rewards.
- *Behavioral capability* are knowledge and skills to enact a behavior.

- *Expectations* refer to what a person thinks may happen based on performing a behavior.
- *Self-efficacy* refers to a person's confidence in their ability to change a behavior.
- *Emotional-coping response* means that people can deal with sources of anxiety or fear that may accompany behavior change.

Motivational interviewing is an approach often used by help-line operators and other professions to help people make changes, especially when people lack the motivation to change on their own (Motivational Interviewing Network of Trainers [MINT], 2021). It is a nonthreatening, collaborative approach that encourages clients to talk about needed change and incorporates good questioning and listening skills that draw out the client's goals and encourage realization about the changes needed to accomplish those goals.

Nikki noted that there typically are not many well-known, public examples of people in long-term recovery. She said, "When you're in the trenches of addiction, you're seeing the worst of the worst, and you might forget your goal, where you're actually headed, but this isn't where you're going to stay."

Nikki was most proud to be affiliated with Consumer Help because of its decades-long commitment to being a peer-run organization. She explained that peers provide a special kind of support because they have been through similar challenges and can be seen as less judgmental and more trustworthy. Peers in recovery also provide hope because they are able to say, "I've been there and I've moved forward." This gives them credibility others may not have. In alignment with the organization's mission, the goal of warmline operators is to get callers to a place where they can visualize themselves in long-term recovery, and that can be done with a good role model.

Like many other warmlines, Consumer Help has realized that keeping calls to 15 minutes once a day helps ensure that multiple callers can get through to an operator. The time limit also helps to keep calls solution- and support-focused. Nikki explained, "If you go too short, you're not effective, but if you go too long, people tend to cycle and say the same thing over and over."

According to their mission statement, "Consumer Help is the organization of people in recovery. We empower others to find their resilience, mental health, and wellness through education, advocacy, and support."

A **mission statement** briefly describes the core purpose of an organization in a way that helps its members keep goals, objectives, and activities on track. It can also reflect values and beliefs. Consumer Help emphasizes the following in their approach to services:

- A **strengths-based approach** to recovery acknowledges that every person, no matter how challenging their situation, has strengths. Identifying those strengths can help people grow. People are more likely to make positive changes when emphasis is on their strengths rather than their deficiencies.
- **Empowerment** is the process of helping a person improve their life situation by increasing their personal, interpersonal, and political power.
- **Resilience** refers to people's ability to adapt and recover from adversity.

GETTING THE WORD OUT ABOUT SERVICES

With the help of the state's funding from the DMHA, as well as other grant funding, Consumer Help covers the costs of employees, rent, supplies, and a small marketing budget. Combined, these grants afford the agency an annual budget of $164,000, which Nikki said is "not a lot, but is sufficient." Because of external funding, the warmline is a free service for callers.

The magnitude of warmline operations can vary widely depending on their scope and funding. For example, Safe Harbor Peer Crisis Services warmline for mental health in Omaha, Nebraska reported answering approximately 12,000 calls a year with an annual budget of $670,000, and the California Peer-Run Warmline answered approximately 28,000 calls/chats in one year on a budget of roughly $3,600,000 (Snibbe, 2019).

A small part of Consumer Help's annual budget is used for marketing the warmline, which includes Nikki's attendance at local conferences and events where she advertises her organization's services to others. At the *Recovery Ride and Rally* (see Chapter 4), for example, she reserved a booth to distribute flyers, brochures, and cards advertising the warmline, as well as pens, bracelets, and stress balls that included the organization's name and contact information. To reserve a booth, Consumer Help donated $100 to the state's Mental Health America affiliate, who granted the organization a space where Nikki could easily interact with attendees.

Consumer Help must convince both callers and the state health department of the value of their warmline service. Promoting the program serves to accrue more callers, or service users, which demonstrates a need for the service and increases the likelihood the state will renew the grant. According to Nikki, the organization currently focuses its resources more on marketing the warmline and other programs and less on fundraising efforts because the current funding from grants is sufficient for their level of programming.

The cost of promotion and marketing efforts must be considered when planning and developing a program budget.

Promotion is the act of communicating the value of a product or service to a specific market or group most likely to benefit.

Marketing is promoting a product or service with the help of research and advertising.

Identifying and communicating directly with every potential person in crisis about the warmline services would be impossible, but Nikki was involved with several community and statewide advisory boards such as the state's Recovery Council, the Mental Health Advisory and Policy Action Committee, and the DMHA policy advisory committee. Her participation creates opportunities to network with others, talk about Consumer Help's services, and promote the warmline, which she enthusiastically embraced. She explained, "Hopefully the information will trickle down because I can't go to every clinic, though I wish I could." She reiterated, "We need the exposure. It gets really important that people understand that we're here."

In Nikki's efforts to network with service providers, she is faced with a common problem. Nikki explained, "We had pretty good name recognition, then it kind of fell off because there's a lot of turnaround in front line staff at the community mental health centers. So, our visibility went away for a bit, and we're trying to build it back up."

High turnover of mental health staff leads to a continual need for agencies to promote their programs. Rates of annual staff turnover in publicly funded mental health organizations are notably high, often ranging from 30% to

60%. Long workdays and lack of support from supervisors contribute to employee burnout in the mental health field (Beidas et al., 2016).

Mental health workers can be at risk of developing **vicarious trauma** due to absorbing the trauma of others, but this condition can be mitigated through awareness and intentional self-care activities.

RECRUITING STAFF AND VOLUNTEERS TO OPERATE THE WARMLINE

Consumer Help, like other warmline operations, is entirely peer-run and is heavily reliant on volunteer operators. All office volunteers and the four paid agency staff self-identify as consumers of mental health services. For many, this includes addiction recovery services.

Agency policy states that 51% of the Consumer Help board of directors, comprised of eight members, must self-identify as consumers of either mental health or addiction recovery services. This means that volunteers, employees, and board members have "been there" and understand mental health and addiction on a personal level.

Nikki uses Consumer Help's *Facebook* page and the nonprofit Association of Peer Recovery Specialists listserv to recruit warmline volunteers. Volunteers must self-identify as being in recovery. The agency also prefers that they have had *Certified Recovery Specialist* (CRS) training, but Nikki noted that they will not be removed from consideration if not. A **certified peer recovery specialist** has lived experience with mental health and/or substance misuse and is formally trained to provide support to others. The certification is valuable because part of the certification process is demonstrating capacity to address one's personal recovery needs and identify healthy boundaries with others.

While it is important that warmline operators have devoted significant time to work through their own mental health and substance use issues, Nikki noted that it is sometimes the volunteers with the most tumultuous histories who excel at doing warmline work. She explained, "Sometimes the more there's been chaos in their lives, and they've learned how to deal with it, the better they are at bringing hope to other people that they can do the same."

Nikki reported that Consumer Help has struggled to retain volunteer operators – in part because the work can be so emotionally demanding. She explained, "We tend to have people who want to volunteer, but they come in, and it's a little too much for them, and they tend not to follow through on it." She recalled, "We've had four potential volunteers do that since I've been Executive Director. They felt like it was just too much for them." Yet, like Nikki, many of the organization's employees began as volunteers. She explained, "Because we're a peer-run organization, and we are so dedicated, we tend to draw dedicated people. The people who work here care deeply about what we do." She added, "That is a big strength of us—our people. I think it's the biggest strength, honestly."

The organizational culture that Nikki described is consistent with a **culture of care** and is commonly found in successful social service organizations. In this type of culture, employees and other contributors are deeply invested in their work because it aligns with their core values (Brody, 2005). At Consumer Help, workers may experience increased job ownership because their job aligns with their personal identities as people in recovery.

The people who work for a program, whether paid or unpaid, are its main resources. They also set the tone for the **organizational culture**, which refers to the values, beliefs, and norms shared within an organization that impact communication and performance expectations.

One disadvantage is that innovation and creativity may be hindered for lack of diverse perspectives.

An advantage of having a distinct organizational culture is that operations have a greater chance of running smoothly because of shared expectations.

Four characteristics tend to increase a workers' sense of job ownership (Dhingra et al., 2021):

- The worker feels that their job serves a *higher purpose* by making a difference in a larger system.
- The worker cares about the people they work with and experiences *emotional bonding* with them.
- The worker enjoys fellowship with co-workers and can *trust* them to contribute to common goals.
- The worker feels *pride in their work* as a result of achieving work tasks that serve a higher cause.

The warmline staff is quite small, with only two full-time and two part-time paid employees. In addition to Nikki's full-time role as Executive Director, one other full-time employee uses half of her time to implement a prison-based program and the other half to answer calls on the warmline.

Nikki said it is difficult to know whether the agency currently has "enough" warmline operators. When callers contact the warmline, they go into a queue and sometimes hang up if their call is not answered right away. Though the warmline tends to be busiest in the early morning, call volume at any time can be unpredictable. Sometimes multiple operators will be available, but there is no caller. Other times, there is only one operator who answers a steady stream of calls during their entire shift. For the most part, Nikki said that the number of calls they take increases with the number of operators they add.

TRAINING WARMLINE OPERATORS AS A PATH TO PROGRAM FIDELITY

Consumer Help has a plan in place for training new warmline volunteers, though the training procedure is largely informal. Volunteer operator trainees have access to a warmline operation packet compiled by the agency. Nikki described the training process as an on-going discussion with the warmline operators about the program goals and what they should and should not do with callers. She and the other more seasoned warmline operators will discuss with new operators what to do if there is a crisis call or any other call inappropriate for the warmline.

Developing a standardized program manual or handbook allows an organization to achieve **program fidelity**, which means they can deliver a program or intervention in the same way regardless of who is implementing it.

This standardization facilitates adherence to shared procedures, policies, and parameters and assists in program evaluation. Without it, evaluators would not know what they are evaluating the program for and how to plan for the evaluation.

With callers' permission, trainees will listen in on phone calls taken by the more experienced operators. Then, they will switch places and act as the operator while someone else listens in. Nikki explained, "We generally have people who are ready to jump in after that training period, but if there's anything they have questions about along the way, or they're just not ready, we can listen in more, or we can have a conversation about what it is that they feel they're lacking."

Mental health organizations, like Consumer Help, must comply with **HIPAA**, the Health Care Insurance Portability Accountability Act, to maintain confidentiality of clients' *personal health information* (PHI). Organizations cannot share PHI with third parties, such as physicians or other service providers, unless clients provide signed authorization.

There are two exceptions to confidentiality:

1. If a service user indicates that they are an imminent danger to themselves or others, the organization is legally bound to inform others of the danger as a duty-to-warn exception.
2. For the purpose of training and supervision, workers within an organization are allowed to communicate with each other about service users in order to improve service delivery.

Otherwise, workers cannot legally discuss service user details outside of a health or mental health organization, or they risk termination and/or legal action. All workers in an organization – whether paid or volunteer – should have a clear understanding of the organization's confidentiality policies.

According to Nikki, warmline operators are trained to step outside of their own recovery experience and focus on what is best for the caller. She sometimes needs to remind operators that interventions that helped them might not necessarily help others – that identifying a successful pathway to recovery depends on the needs and experiences of the individual (Kelly et al., 2017). Being a warmline operator does not mean that you tell people what to do. "That's a recipe for disaster!" she emphasized. Instead, callers have their own journeys, and warmline operators are present to offer support during that journey.

EVALUATING PROGRAM SUCCESS WITH THE HELP OF A LOGIC MODEL

How successful is the warmline? Consumer Help has kept years of call log data in hard copy, which can be analyzed more closely if ever needed. However, Nikki, chuckling to herself, admitted, "We have so much data that is being collected, but we don't know what to do with it yet."

Nikki tipped her glasses downward and pulled out a document with geometric shapes, arrows, and boxes. "This is a logic model for our organization," she stated. "Basically, if we have these resources and do these activities, we should expect these results. It's a series of 'if this. . .then this' statements." During her time at Consumer Help, Nikki had participated in several trainings about creating logic models to assist with program planning. The structure provided by a logic model made sense to her because, in her experience, "scope creep" can happen when organizations feel too ambitious or get pulled in another direction from their mission and original objectives. In one logic model training, she was asked to write down all the components of her program on different sticky notes, organize the notes, and draw arrows with a dry erase marker among the sticky notes to depict how they related to each other.

Logic models are graphic depictions used to describe relationships among resources, program activities, outputs, and desired outcomes (Centers for Disease Control [CDC], 2018). In general, logic models possess four components:

- *Inputs* are the resources that are needed to plan, implement, and evaluate a program. They include human resources, partnerships, funding sources, equipment, supplies, materials, space, gifts, etc.
- *Activities* are the interventions, curriculum, or other strategies used to promote behavior change.
- *Outputs* focus on the scope and process of the activities, such as number of participants attending an event, the number of students in a class, the number of workshops hosted, the amount of information distributed or disseminated, or the number of partnerships formed, etc.
- *Outcomes* are changes that occur because of the activities and outputs. They are divided into short-term (e.g. changes in awareness, attitudes, knowledge, skills), mid-term (e.g. changes in behavior or environment), and long-term results (e.g. health status, quality of life, and morbidity and mortality indicators).

A logic model should illustrate how each activity leads to certain outputs that then lead to certain outcomes that ultimately indicate whether a program is successful in meeting its overall mission.

Propping her glasses back, Nikki emphasized the importance of keeping the organization's mission statement and program goals in mind when planning a public health program. Nikki explained, "While someone might be excited about implementing a new or trendy activity, it needs to logically tie back to the program's goals. You have to think about the sequence, too." She added, "What's the logical order, what must be implemented before something else can be implemented?"

In Nikki's case, as Executive Director, she had to acquire the necessary inputs needed to implement the program activities: human resources like hiring and training staff, infrastructure like the phone lines, internet connection, headsets, computers, and other equipment – even the office space itself and grant funding to facilitate purchases. She needed to plan time for recruiting, hiring, and training staff, being sure they practice and prepare to independently take calls. This would make it possible for operators to effectively receive and respond to the phone calls and offer peer support, which were considered activities within the logic of the program. She also had to make sure staff receive regular continuing education on techniques, such as motivational interviewing.

The next step, she noted, is to consider the relevant outputs of the program activities. "I break it down really simply," she said. "Basically, our outputs are the number of people who have spoken to one of our warmline staff." Nikki refered to this **metric** as "monthly call frequency."

Nikki discussed how at the end of every call, warmline operators at Consumer Help complete call logs that are then stored in hard copy in the agency's office and electronically within their computer database. The call log includes the following information for each caller:

- Name (if the caller wants to share it)
- Date
- Call start and end time
- Operator name
- Area code
- How they heard about the warmline
- Whether they are a first-time caller

The agency uses these logs to track the number of warmline calls received per month. Then, based on these records, they "bill" (i.e. generate and send invoices) to the state's DMHA, which then triggers the release of state grant money provided to Consumer Help for operation costs.

Monthly call frequency is an important metric for Consumer Help. But Nikki asserted that the most meaningful data is whether any changes take place in the callers' lives as a result of the warmline. Referring to her "if this. . .then this" strategy, she illustrated, "If my staff are taking calls in the ways they've been trained, then callers may gain a new perspective that helps them keep going for another day, they might make a significant life change, such as drawing a new boundary with a toxic friend or family member. The callers may even decide to take a step toward quitting substances, such as getting treatment. The support we offer here can change a life, even if it's just an attitude change."

Some warmlines aim to demonstrate a reduction in 911 calls and hospital visits by providing pre-crisis support to callers. But, is it really possible to verify why something *does not* happen? Nikki lamented, "How can we possibly know for sure that a person would have gone into crisis if they *hadn't* called the warmline? Maybe we can never know for sure." Nikki and other stakeholders want to know whether warmline services are making a positive impact in their community, but determining whether the warmline program impacts long-term outcomes can be particularly difficult.

Nonetheless, additional information in the call log, if the caller is willing to disclose it, can begin to capture this data:

- Reason for the call
- Shared peer experience
- Where they would have sought help if not for the warmline
- Helpfulness of the call, on a scale of 1–10

Nikki has hope that they will eventually have the resources to hire a professional program evaluator who can dig deeper into the many years of call log data that Consumer Help has stored. Only then will they truly observe the extent to which their services are helping the community.

One of the first comprehensive assessments of a peer-run warmline was conducted for Warmline Inc, in Milwaukee, WI. At the time, Warmline Inc. had been in operation for 10 years, received over 50,000 calls, and trained 110 volunteer peer counselors as warmline operators. With the help of a local foundational grant, the organization hired an external evaluator to lead process, formative, and cost-effectiveness evaluations (Stephens, 2019).

Process Evaluation

From call logs, researchers learned basic descriptive information about the warmline's daily operation or processes, which included outputs. From this data, evaluators were able to describe who was accessing services and how they were delivered:

- They found that the warm line was receiving an average of 550 calls per month and 22 calls per night.
- They also learned that the operators generally did a good job of following the policy of limiting calls to 15 minutes – 80% of calls were 15 minutes or less, and the majority of the remaining calls did not exceed 20 minutes.
- Additionally, they learned that 97% of callers were repeat callers, and 60% were women.
- Moreover, less than 1% of calls could be considered "hot calls," meaning that callers were in crisis rather than pre-crisis stage.

Formative Evaluation

A member of the research team also interviewed eight consistent warmline users who were identified by operators and agreed to participate in the evaluation. The callers were asked how they became aware of the warmline, why they continued to use it, and what could be improved:

- Callers expressed gratitude in being able to talk with someone who had similar challenges in a safe, anonymous, and non-stigmatizing setting.
- They also liked that most operators offered ideas and made suggestions but did not typically deliver heavy-handed advice.
- They understood the need for a 15-minute call limit and preferred that the warmline establish a queue where they could wait for an operator rather than having to call back repeatedly.
- Callers also noted that they sometimes interacted better with some operators than others.

A member of the research team also reached out to social service professionals and asked them to reflect on the warmline. Some professionals expressed concern about lack of clinical training for peer operators and suggested that more training for operators might help credibility. They also stated that extended nighttime hours for the warmline might enhance its impact, yet they recognized that availability of funding was a limitation.

Cost-Effectiveness Evaluation

Results of the cost-effectiveness analysis indicated that warmline services were cost-effective:

- The estimated cost of one warmline call to their clinic was $10, whereas the estimated cost of one 911 call was $100 and a trip to the emergency room was $700.
- From this data, the study determined that the warmline program saved the state roughly $4.8 million per year, not accounting for other cost-saving benefits, such as providing an assistive tool cost-free to police and mental health providers who regularly refer people and clients to the warmline.

Outcomes associated with behavioral and mental health changes in warmline users were not part of this evaluation, but data regarding such outcomes would be ideal to have when evaluating the overall impact of the program.

DISCUSSION QUESTIONS

1. What are the benefits in using peers as facilitators? What might be some downsides to look for or precautions to take?

2. If you were trying to convince a donor to support a warmline program, what would you use in your "sales pitch"?

3. Think about the importance of creating visibility for this type of program. What types of strategies would catch your attention?

4. Think about the challenges of measuring the impact of this program. Would an increase in monthly calls be a sign that the program is working or that the program is failing? Explain.

5. Consider the different ways a peer-run warmline program could evaluated. What is the benefit of talking to those who use the program? What is the benefit of talking to service providers?

6. What type of "scope creep" might occur if a program is not following its original logic model? Can you think of a real-life example when a program began to offer a service outside of its original mission?

ACTIVITIES

1. Imagine you are creating a warmline program for one of the following: (1) parents who are at risk of abusing their children, (2) adults who self-soothe through overeating and are struggle with their health, or (3) adolescents who struggle to avoid giving into negative peer pressure (e.g. to skip school, vandalize, steal). Address the following:
   - What are the goals of your program?
   - Will you use peer facilitators? Why or why not?
   - If you use peer facilitators, how would you recruit them? What special training might they need? If you do not use peer facilitators, who will you use?
   - How will you make the public aware of this new resource?
   - How can this program use a strengths-based perspective?

2. Imagine you are creating a program to educate school-aged children about the misuse of prescription medication, resisting peer pressure to use drugs, or engaging in prosocial behavior conducive to healthy living. Include the following and be prepared to explain the logic for their inclusion:

- 5 inputs you would need to implement the rest of the model
- 3 activities
- 3 outputs
- 2 short or mid-range outcomes
- 1 long-term outcome
- Arrows indicating how all of the above are connected.

REFERENCES

Bandura, A. (1977). *Social Learning Theory*. Englewood Cliffs, NJ: Prentice Hall.

Bandura, A. (1986). *Social Foundations of Thought and Action*. Englewood Cliffs, NJ: Prentice Hall.

Beidas, R. S., Marcus, S., Wolk, C. B., Powell, B., Aarons, G. A., Evans, A. C., Hurford, M. O., Hadley, T., Adams, D. R., Walsh, L. M., Babbar, S., Barg, F., & Mandell, D. S. (2016). A prospective examination of clinician and supervisor turnover within the context of implementation of evidence-based practices in a publicly-funded mental health system. *Administration and Policy in Mental Health*, *43*(5), 640–649. https://doi.org/10.1007/s10488015-0673-6

Brody, R. (2005). *Effectively Managing Human Service Organizations* (3rd ed.). Thousand Oaks, CA: Sage.

Centers for Disease Control (CDC) (2018). *Program Evaluation Framework Checklist for Step 2*. https://www.cdc.gov/evaluation/steps/step2/index.htm

Dhingra, N., Samo, A., Schaninger, B., & Schrimper, M. (2021). *Help Your Employees Find Purpose–Or Watch Them Leave*. McKinsey & Company. https://www.mckinsey.com/capabilities/people-and-organizationalperformance/our-insights/help-your-employees-find-purpose-or-watch-them-leave#.

Kelly, J.F., Bergman, B., Hoeppner, B.B., Vilsaint, C., & White, W. (2017). Prevalence and pathways of recovery from drug and alcohol problems in the US population: Implications for practice, research, and policy. *Drug and Alcohol Dependence*, *181*(1), 162–169.

Motivational Interviewing Network of Trainers (MINT) (2021). MI information and training. https://motivationalinterviewing.org/

Rotter, J. (1954). *Social Learning and Clinical Psychology*. New York: Prentice Hall.

Stephens, S. (2019). It's not a hotline, it's a 'warmline': It gives mental health help before a crisis heats up. *USA Today/Kaiser Health News*. https://www.usatoday.com/story/news/health/2019/12/04/mental-health-warmlines-not-hotlines-help-before-crisis/2600402001/

Snibbe, K. (2019). What you can and cannot expect from California's new mental health line: The state is spending $10.8 million over three years on the project. *East Bay Times/Southern California News Group*. https://www.eastbaytimes.com/2019/10/11/what-you-can-and-cannot-expect-from-californias-new-mental-health-line/

CHAPTER

AN INTERPROFESSIONAL SYMPOSIUM

RECRUITING PLANNING COMMITTEE MEMBERS AND SETTING MEASURABLE GOALS AND OBJECTIVES

In this chapter, we share the experience of a planning committee dedicated to taking an interprofessional and collaborative approach to substance use disorder prevention in their region. They plan an inaugural, community-wide symposium on substance use issues, bringing together a variety of voices and resources. They learn from this experience about creating detailed objectives that assist with planning and evaluation.

Ten minutes into the meeting, a group of professionals huddled over the table, fiddling with the video conference microphone and cursing the technology. The group was holding an initial planning meeting to

Health Promotion Planning: Learning from the Accounts of Public Health Practitioners,
First Edition. Jean Marie S. Place, Jonel Thaller, and Scott S. Hall.
© 2024 John Wiley & Sons, Inc. Published 2024 by John Wiley & Sons, Inc.

address substance misuse in their county. The meeting organizer, Jenna Foster, was having trouble figuring out how to flip the volume from the monitor – where a colleague's image was broadcast in real time – to the microphone, so that everyone around the table could hear her speak. The microphone lay dormant in the center of the boardroom table. Jenna gave up using the microphone and everyone scooted their seats closer to the 72-in. monitor suspended on the wall, heads cocked toward the screen to hear words that sounded muffled and somewhat muted, as if the conversation were traveling through a wind tunnel. They did their best to follow along with what their remote colleague was saying, despite the less-than-ideal tech situation.

As the Director of Interprofessional Development at the local university, Jenna had brought this group of local professionals together to discuss possible projects to address the rising toll of opioid misuse in the community. After introductions, they went around the table and shared observations and opinions. What could they do to address substance misuse in their community that did not require external grant funding or large installments of money? What was within their expertise? What did the community need the most?

Programs begin in a variety of ways. Some programs begin organically when there is an obvious need in the community and consensus about the type of programming needed. Other times, community-wide needs assessments are necessary to identify and prioritize programmatic gaps (see Chapter 1). Still other times, grant sponsors dictate what they are willing to fund and program planners respond with programs that fit the predetermined criteria of the sponsor's **RFP** or "request for proposals" on a specific topic.

ASSEMBLING A PLANNING COMMITTEE

A few weeks prior to this first tech-challenged gathering, Jenna initiated an email thread to invite colleagues to form a planning committee. She began by introducing two colleagues whom she felt would work well together but who had different but complementary specialties within the field of addictions. Both worked in the addictions sphere, one as a project manager for a state-wide hospital network and the other for a criminal justice-based nonprofit organization. Jenna then asked both women to invite additional professionals from within different sub-specialties of addictions into the conversation. They did, and their group expanded to five members.

One can form a planning committee by simply inviting or recruiting people to serve. Recruitment can also occur through marketing and publicity, such as advertising via a newsletter or social media site. Other common means of forming a committee include holding an election, making formal appointments, or initiating an application process.

Intentionally inviting an interprofessional group of people to serve on a committee or panel is an important way to broaden community input and buy-in.

A formal email invitation to participate on a committee or panel should include an opening salutation with the intended recipient's correct name and title. The sender should begin the communication by introducing themselves if they are unknown to the recipient, then follow with a clear and direct request. The information provided in the invitation should be detailed enough that the recipient knows what is being asked of them, but not so detailed with irrelevant information that the recipient is confused, irritated, or overwhelmed. The sender should avoid jargon or vague phrasing and only use exclamation marks sparingly. A professional closing should encourage the recipient to reach out if they have any questions about the request. A signature line with the sender's contact information should conclude the message.

This small, interprofessional group of addictions-related practitioners formed the planning committee for a community-wide symposium focused on substance use disorders. During this first meeting, as the group continued to grapple with glitches in technology, the discussion moved toward how they might build an interprofessional panel of state and local practitioners to share expertise with symposium attendees, which would include practitioners, concerned community members, and university students. The group members brainstormed potential avenues to bring interdisciplinary experts to the university's campus, while also ensuring that the event would have a townhall-feel, geared toward addressing the questions that students and local practitioners might have. After a robust discussion about whom to invite to the panel, Jenna created a shared account accessible through the Internet where the group could store planning documents. Though the first meeting was marred with technology trouble, everyone left with energy and excitement. After the initial meeting, the group began to meet bi-weekly (every two weeks) to plan the symposium.

As they later reflected on additional people who could be added to the planning committee to enhance the planning process, they realized that, in the rush to generate an event idea and grab anyone who could help, they had failed to think strategically about who should be at the table. This core group had inadvertently omitted students from the planning process, even though they were important stakeholders in the event and the event would be held on campus. Despite the oversight, the planning committee was comprised of two professors. They could potentially represent the needs of their students, although only from a secondhand perspective. This omission was a glaring oversight.

Partnering with a variety of organizations and respected individuals in a community means that more resources are at the group's disposal to use toward the event, the hands of more stakeholders help lift the burden of planning the event, and there is greater access to the ideas and expertise of diverse people and organizations.

Diverse and inclusive membership on planning committees have important benefits: committee members have increased feelings of program ownership and they can help spread support of the program, as well as providing insights on program development. Ultimately, an inclusive planning committee can help make programs more impactful for the people that need it.

Research indicates that teams with more diverse knowledge and ethnic backgrounds tend to be more creative (Hundschell et al., 2022), though diverse perspectives can also make it more difficult to create group consensus around a plan of action (Harvey, 2013). Being able to cultivate trust and validation within a team can enhance diverse groups' abilities to maximize the benefits of having multiple perspectives.

Fortunately, the committee varied in terms of race, age, gender, and professional discipline, and also included people in recovery. One of the original planning committee members, Juli Kohl, had insider's knowledge into substance misuse. In addition to her role as Deputy Director for a mental and behavioral health nonprofit, she was in long-term recovery from a substance use disorder. Juli was unique in that she possessed knowledge as an "informant" and also as a "respondent." Because of her professional role and years of education and training, she was an **informant** who could provide an expert's *informed* opinion on, for example, the pros and cons of specific evidence-based interventions available to people in recovery. However, because of her life experience as a person in recovery, she was also a **respondent** who could *respond* with insight into how to best support a person in recovery.

Juli also used her lived experience to ensure that promotional materials for the event modeled empowering language for those impacted by addiction. **Person-first language** centers the humanity of a person experiencing an issue rather than the specific disease, disorder, or condition. For example, using the term "person in recovery" (rather than "recovering addict") indicates that the person is a human *first* and is not defined solely by their struggles. Juli knew firsthand the shame that can come from being labeled an "addict." With those years behind her, she wanted to give back to the community by spreading hope rather than shame.

McKenzie et al. (2017) emphasizes that a planning committee should have a combination of "doers" and "influencers." **Doers** are people who can "roll up their sleeves" and get physical work done to make sure the program is planned and implemented properly. **Influencers** wield authority so that "with a single phone call" they can rally resources or generate support from others. Without a mixture of both types, committees might burn out doing all the work themselves, or spin their wheels waiting for others to step up and move the project forward.

PLANNING COMMITTEE IN ACTION

Over the next six months, the committee planned the county's first-ever Symposium on Substance Use Disorders. The group seemed especially productive because they shared the "doer" load equally – nobody deemed themselves too important to spend time crafting and editing the digital invitations, reserving rooms, or organizing speaker schedules. Given her role as a member of the Dean's University Leadership Team, Jenna acted as an influencer by requesting the support of the University Provost who provided a welcome to attendees at the symposium. However, like the rest of the team, Jenna was also a doer. She was the de-facto leader who took notes on action items, kept the meetings to one hour, reviewed what had been accomplished from meeting to meeting, and maintained discussion centered around main points in the agenda before moving to new discussion items. These strategies made for well-organized and smoothly run meetings. She also took meeting minutes, which included a review of who attended each meeting and what was talked about, including next steps and issues tabled for discussion at later meetings.

Planning committee members leveraged resources from their organizational affiliations to make the event happen. For example,

Tony Bianchi was involved in a state-wide initiative to train rural healthcare providers on opioid use disorder. Juli's mental and behavioral health nonprofit was a subsidiary organization of the well-known Mental Health America. Juli's and Tony's affiliations meant the group had access to their membership email lists, which were used to spread the word about the event. Juli reflected, "I promoted the event with people at work because I was excited to help the event take place." She recalled, "We even got the Executive Director to give the keynote address!" The benefit of those connections was directly related to the powerful resources the planning committee members had at their disposal.

The group began to coalesce around the idea of hosting two consecutive panels at the symposium: one with state experts and the other with local experts. "We felt like local voices needed to be heard and highlighted, but we also wanted to know what was going on outside of our area. And, we wanted all of these conversations to happen in a townhall-sort of way," one of the planning committee members explained. The panelists would act as **key informants**, people who have the knowledge and expertise to report on the needs of those they represent.

Key informants can provide a birds-eye view of issues while also cutting to the heart of an issue and identifying what needs to be done.

While key informants are often experts in their field, they still bring biases with them. Because they represent only one perspective, it is important to couple data from key informants with other primary and secondary data to form a more complete picture of the needs in a community.

KEEPING AN EYE ON THE MISSION, GOALS, AND OBJECTIVES

Each time the planning committee met to develop the symposium, they reminded each other of their primary purpose: to promote the importance of *interprofessional practice* in addressing substance misuse. They drafted the symposium's mission statement accordingly: "The symposium will focus on interprofessional and collaborative approaches to substance use disorder prevention, detection, treatment, and recovery."

The committee's selection of panelists intentionally joined together representatives of different fields to model the collaborative nature of prevention, detection, treatment, and recovery. They also referred to the mission statement when they developed questions to ask the panelists. They wanted panelists' answers to elucidate how interprofessional practice worked in application. They also kept the mission statement in mind when they advertised the program. They reached across disciplinary silos to publicize the event across campus, emphasizing relevant content for a range of professions. They aimed to have the promotion of interdisciplinary practice influence all the choices they made throughout the planning process.

Program **goals** work in tandem with a mission statement, specifying what will change because of the program and who it will affect. Goals are broad targets the program sets out to accomplish. Goals should start with action verbs, such as improve, strengthen, promote, increase, minimize, prevent, etc. (CDC, n.d.). Goals are action-oriented, indicate the direction of impact, and provide guidance on what planners should focus on.

Specific **objectives** are typically a set of steps that "break down the goals into smaller parts" and create "measurable actions by which the goal can be accomplished" (CDC, n.d.).

Objectives, goals, and mission statements are all interconnected; when objectives are met, goals can be achieved, thereby fulfilling the program's mission. Each objective should address what will change, how much change will take place, when the change will occur, and among whom the change will occur.

Objectives that promote change in a target population can be classified as impact objectives or outcome objectives.

- *Impact objectives* aim for immediate effects of the program among the target population, such as changes in awareness, knowledge, attitudes, skills, behaviors, or the economic, physical, political, service or psychosocial environments. These objectives could be parallel to "short-term outcomes" or "mid-term outcomes" contained in logic models (see Chapter 7).
- *Outcome objectives* aim for long-term changes in health status among the target population, such as disability, morbidity and mortality, or quality of life indicators. These objectives could be parallel to "long-term outcomes" contained in logic models (see Chapter 7).

The planning committee set goals for the symposium that mirrored the US Department of Health and Human Services' strategy for addressing the opioid crisis:

1. Improve access to treatment and recovery services
2. Strengthen the understanding of the epidemic through better public health surveillance
3. Promote use of overdose-reversing drugs

The committee viewed the symposium as contributing, albeit in a minor way, toward reaching the broad U.S. goals. When asked to reflect on the objectives set for the symposium, Jenna hung her head. "We're going to change things around for next year and do our objectives better the next time." The biggest change, she said, would be creating specific objectives that could be more easily evaluated. She laughed good-naturedly, "What good are objectives if you can't measure them?"

Ideally, symposium objectives should describe what specific changes would occur among attendees, when those changes would occur, and how the changes would be achieved. For example, one of the original objectives stated:

■ "Discuss what community agencies in the region are doing to address the opioid crisis."

The original objective lacked measurable criteria to be a well-written impact objective. As written, the objective did not describe who would be affected and what success would look like.

The previously vague objective could be revised to be more easily measurable and time-bound:

■ "By the end of the symposium on 14 March, at least 90% of attendees will be able to list in an exit survey one program in the region with treatment and recovery services."

The revised objective is specific and measurable enough to be evaluated in a concrete manner and help determine the success of the symposium. To meet the objective, the planning committee could request that each panel presenter describe at least one addictions-related service with which they are affiliated and provide additional information via flyers or agency swag – whatever it takes to increase the chances that symposium attendees will remember at least one service. This is an **impact objective** because it is focuses on increasing awareness among attendees.

Another somewhat vague objective stated:

■ "Conduct a Naloxone training for students, faculty, and other interested community members"

Although this objective aligned with the broad U.S. goal to "promote the use of overdose-reversing drugs," it too lacked detail sufficient to be measurable. As written, it is not known what will change, how much change will take place, or when the change will occur. If a training is held and only two people show up, should it be considered a success? Specific criteria are needed to dictate what attainment of the objective would look like:

The objective could be revised to state:

- "By the end of the training on 14 March, at least 20 people (students, faculty members, and/or community members) will have attended a Naloxone training."

Additional impact objectives could be created to articulate what could be gained from the training, including increased knowledge, awareness, or skills. Instead of simply "attending" a training, the objective could be re-written to outline that people would be able to list three actions that need to take place to reverse an overdose, or that people could list three symptoms of an overdose like blue lips, unresponsiveness, and shallow breathing.

Another objective also lacked sufficient information and was too vague for measuring success:

- "Recognize the interprofessional approach and skills required to address the opioid addiction crisis."

The impact objective could be revised to state:

- "In a post-test survey, attendees will report an increase of 10% from baseline on their knowledge of how to use interprofessional practice to address the opioid crisis."

In this case, it would be important to assess participants on their knowledge of interprofessional practice prior to attending the symposium as well as after the symposium to determine whether participants' knowledge had increased.

When crafting objectives, it is important to adhere to the **SMART guidelines** for writing objectives.

- Is the objective **S**pecific? This means that the objective specifies who the target population is for a specific activity or action.
- Is it **M**easurable? This means that the objective specifies a detectable change expected due to the activity or action.
- Is it **A**chievable? This means the objective can be reasonably accomplished in a context of given resources.
- Is it **R**elevant? This means the objective clearly addresses the targeted problem.
- Is it **T**ime-phased? This means the objective includes a timeline for when the action or activity will be completed.

THE FRUITS OF PLANNING

Two months prior to the symposium date, the committee was pleased to learn that all their email invitations to prospective panelists had been accepted. They were especially proud of the work they had done to identify and connect with interdisciplinary practitioners at the state level even though their event was still new:

- A state representative for the National Alliance of Recovery Residencies would speak on the need for sober-living housing after intensive inpatient or outpatient treatment services and barriers to recruiting landlords to sponsor recovery housing.
- A physician who worked in a nearby county and who had been interviewed several times on National Public Radio (NPR) would share his experience treating the youngest victims of the opioid epidemic – those with neonatal withdrawal syndrome – and speak about state-level policies related to medication-assisted treatment (MAT).
- A university professor and licensed social worker who had become the leading expert on trauma-informed care in the state would emphasize the importance of trauma-informed, recovery-oriented behavioral health services, especially for people struggling with substance use disorder.
- A representative from the state organization responsible for training and certifying peer recovery coaches would speak about the value of peer-led services (see Chapter 7) and new trends in peer recovery coaching and billing through Medicaid.
- A state healthcare leader would speak on barriers to creating new addiction services. As a long-time healthcare administrator, she possessed a uniquely detailed understanding of local, state, and federal policies that could positively or negatively affect treatment efforts for opioid use disorder.

The presenter line-up for the local panel was equally impressive and diverse in sub-specialty areas:

- Darby Montegro from the local Coordinating Council on Substance Use Prevention (CCSUP) would discuss the successes of the youth team (see Chapter 5), while also recognizing that the team was not evidence-based and was only one part of the public health intervention puzzle. She would discuss gaps in prevention programming within the local school district and ways that stakeholders from the community could help address them.
- The director of a local women's recovery center had been invited in hopes she could humanize the story of addiction and recovery on behalf of the many patients she saw as a behavioral health

psychologist. As someone approaching retirement, she would discuss the knowledge and wisdom she had gained throughout her career.

- The CEO of the local federally qualified health center (FQHC) would share about the need for stakeholders to communicate more consistently and bridge silos that artificially create information-sharing barriers.

On the day of the event, the planning committee met the panelists, guests, and attendees with elbow bumps instead of handshakes. It was the very early days of the pandemic, before many institutions retreated to virtual communication platforms, and there was a lot of uncertainty as to whether one should wear a mask, how long viruses can live on surfaces, and what a super-spreader event was. People streamed into the conference room, very few wearing masks and some doing fist bumps instead of elbow bumps. Despite the uncertainty about what this new epidemic would mean for the community, most seats in the room remained filled throughout the four-hour symposium, suggesting there was abundant interest in the topic.

USING TECHNOLOGY TO GATHER FEEDBACK FROM EVENT PARTICIPANTS

Symposium attendees preregistered for the event using an online platform. Upon registration, attendees were asked to indicate whether they were interested in receiving updates about a community coalition focused on addressing the local substance use crisis. The data collected from the online registration platform indicated that most attendees were indeed interested. By asking registrants to indicate their interest in forming a coalition, the planning committee had strategically begun to create a registry of contact information for professionals and organizations who could help respond to the addiction crisis in their region.

Additionally, at the end of the event, on a PowerPoint slide displayed at the front of the room, a black and white QR code appeared for attendees to provide feedback on features of the event. Based on a 10-point Likert scale, attendees could assess their satisfaction with the location of the event, the ease of transportation/parking, and the length of the event. The committee already knew that there was general discontent with the limited parking on campus. However, the data collected could confirm this anecdotal evidence. Attendees could also indicate other changes they would like to see in future symposiums. This data is useful for creating process objectives next year focused on improving communication, availability, and access to parking.

Impact and outcome objectives are different from process objectives. **Process objectives** outline what the planning committee needs to do to carry out the program as planned. Process objectives include daily and weekly activities for planners to do as part of program preparation, implementation, and evaluation. Process objectives are connected to process evaluation (see Chapters 4 and 7) – process objectives relate to planning the program and process evaluation relates to analyzing the planning process afterward.

At the closing of the symposium, Jenna approached the mic and spoke to the room full of engaged attendees. She noted that their registration responses indicated strong community support for an interprofessional coalition to address addiction issues in the county. With undeniable excitement in her voice, Jenna called upon the people in the room to keep an eye out for more announcements and invitations to coalition building activities. She encouraged the attendees to view the symposium as the kick-off event for a more long-term effort to combat substance use disorder in the community.

After many months of brainstorming, planning, and then finally implementation, the planning committee was thrilled with the way the symposium had gone that day, but also exhausted. Offering a sigh of relief that their work was finally over for that day, they would soon regroup to do it all again.

DISCUSSION QUESTIONS

1. What type of online meeting technologies have you used? What were the advantages or disadvantages of each? Describe how you typically address tech challenges. How might using new technologies impact the planning process for better or worse?

2. How well do you think professors can represent the needs of students? What needs do you think they are aware of and which needs are they not? What might a student bring to the table at a planning committee for opioid intervention that a professor could not?

3. If you were asked to be part of a planning committee, whose voices and interests might you represent? What voices and interests would you need to be made aware of?

4. Why might diverse backgrounds on a team result in greater creativity? What potential challenges might emerge because of this diversity? How can challenges be overcome?

5. Why would it be important to have a member of the symposium planning committee be someone who had been in long-term recovery?

6. Think of any event in which you have participated – whether a community volunteer effort, high school prom, or a family vacation. Who were the doers and who were the influencers? Why? Consider your family or a group of friends – when you plan an outing or get-together, are you more often to take the doer or influencer role? Why?

7. Why might people hesitate to create clear objectives for their goals? What can make objectives difficult to create?

8. What do you think of the revised versions of the three objectives discussed above? Can you refine them any further?

9. What outcome objectives could result from the symposium over time?

ACTIVITIES

1. Pretend that you are the project manager for a local food drive program, and you would like to introduce your volunteer coordinator to a school principal. Write a sample introductory email using the suggestions provided in the narrative above.

2. Gauge the current diversity of your classroom and note the voices and interests that may be missing.

3. Look up online templates for taking meeting minutes and observe how the templates compare and contrast. What is most helpful from these templates?

4. Imagine you are part of an organization whose mission it is to end childhood hunger in an area. Create at least two different goals that align with this mission. For each goal, create at least one process objective, one impact objective, and one outcome objective.

REFERENCES

Centers for Disease Control (CDC) (n.d.) *Developing Program Goals and Measurable Objectives*. https://www.cdc.gov/std/program/pupestd/developing%20program%20goals%20and%20objectives.pdf

Harvey, S. (2013). A different perspective: The multiple effects of deep level diversity on group creativity. *Journal of Experimental Social Psychology*, 49(5), 822–832. https://doi.org/10.1016/j.jesp.2013.04.004

Hundschell, A., Razinskas, S., Backmann, J., & Hoegl, M. (2022). The effects of diversity on creativity: A literature review and synthesis. *Psychologie Appliquee [Applied Psychology]*, 71(4), 1598–1634. https://doi.org/10.1111/apps.12365

McKenzie, J., Neiger, B., & Thackeray, R. (2017). *Planning, Implementing, and Evaluating Health Promotion Programs: A Primer*. USA: Pearson.

CHAPTER

9

RECOVERY CAFÉ

BUILDING AN ENVIRONMENTAL CHANGE STRATEGY FOR POSITIVE HEALTH OUTCOMES

In this chapter, we explore the process of initiating environmental change in a community through the hosting of a Recovery Café - a welcoming location that is open, free, and safe for people recovering from substance use disorders. Program planning is successful when communities are engaged in building these kinds of spaces.

Outside of a nondescript church building downtown, a plastic A-frame sign on the sidewalk announces the presence of a Recovery Café. The sign includes the Café's logo and says, "Welcome to Recovery Café! Please Enter Here."

Meals are served at the Recovery Café, but do not be confused – it is not a restaurant. The title is intended to evoke imagery of a lighthearted public space where people gather for refreshments and conversation. But, unlike a typical café, people can mingle at the Recovery Café without spending any money. The Recovery Café is a free space where

Health Promotion Planning: Learning from the Accounts of Public Health Practitioners,
First Edition. Jean Marie S. Place, Jonel Thaller, and Scott S. Hall.

members and guests can eat a meal, attend a workshop or sober social activity, participate in a Recovery Circle, meet with a certified peer recovery coach, or just hang out in the common area and play cards or work on a jigsaw puzzle. Rose Staybrite, the Executive Director, described the purpose succinctly, "Recovery Café is a space where members can go to be seen, known, and loved for who they are and where they are in their journey through life."

As a national nonprofit organization, Recovery Café Network facilitates the development of open and affirming recovery support communities where social and educational activities take place in a drug- and alcohol-free space (Recovery Café Network, 2017).

The Recovery Café model welcomes members who are in recovery from any type of addiction or maladaptive situation. Even if they have not been addicted to substances, many people develop unhealthy habits of coping that manifest as addiction to things like sensation, approval, control, security, and suffering. Like an addiction to substances, these addictions can also be quite difficult to break.

The Recovery Café philosophy is that "everyone is in recovery from something" – they may be in recovery from illicit drug or alcohol use, but they also might be in recovery from domestic abuse, homelessness, grief, news of a chronic illness, codependency, or even perfectionism. The purpose of each localized Café is to foster a love-based, peer recovery community that supports members in their recovery from any barrier that prevents them from living a fulfilling life.

Built upon a belief that each person is worthy of love regardless of their past circumstances, the Recovery Café model encourages members to connect with the love within themselves and others, with the message that "your life matters."

Rose, an athletic woman in her 30s, wore a T-shirt and jogging shoes to work each day. She was animated as she talked about the basic premise for Recovery Café.

"As human beings, we're wired to bond with others, and when we're unable to do so, we may use other means to find the same sort of comfort and satisfaction that bonding provides," she explained. "If disconnection is often the catalyst for addiction, it makes sense to me that connection will be part of the solution." She added, "I know focusing on connection could be considered simplistic since we know that heroin and other opiates are highly addictive and that they affect brain chemistry, but I love thinking of connection as one of the important remedies for addiction."

> In his best-selling book, *Chasing the Scream*, Johann Hari (2015) suggested that the cure for addiction is connection. He noted a series of experiments conducted by Canadian psychologist Bruce Alexander where lab rats were isolated in a bare cage and given the option of drinking either regular water or heroin water. The rats became addicted to the heroin water and eventually died from consuming it. In contrast, rats who resided in a more comfortable cage, stocked with treats and playthings and accompanied by other rats, did not regularly seek out or become addicted to the heroin water. Presumably they chose not to drink it because they were more interested in the variety of other activities available to them.

Recovery Café knows the value of connection. When a visitor approached the check-in desk just inside the building's entryway, a volunteer warmly greeted the man by name. Volunteers – referred to as Café Companions – act as attentive hosts, circulating the common area, welcoming visitors, and making friendly conversation.

"Radical hospitality" is at the core of the Café, where genuine warmth and inclusivity is intended to override shame, ego, and other barriers that thwart human connection. **Radical hospitality** means noticing and acknowledging who needs special attention, introducing yourself and learning other peoples' names, and taking the time to learn what is meaningful to each person. The Recovery Café's tag line states, "Community is brewing!" and members often enact radical hospitality over a cup of coffee.

In the Café's main meeting room, Rose pointed out a woman who was playing *Uno* with a Café Companion at one of the large tables. "She was so skittish when she first arrived, very avoidant," Rose remembered. She acknowledged that people in recovery can spend a lifetime managing their disorder, and they may progress through recovery in a nonlinear manner at different rates and using various strategies. The woman playing *Uno* smiled tentatively when she beat her opponent at a round of the card game. Rose commented how the woman had withdrawn from opioids alone in a jail cell. When she was released from incarceration, there were no formal residential treatment services available to her. "No sober living housing," Rose said. "No treatment center. But there was the Recovery Café. We can't do it all, but we fill in the gaps where we can."

The Recovery Café is an example of an environmental change strategy for health promotion.

An **environmental change strategy** involves changing the economic, social, or physical surroundings or contexts that affect health outcomes. According to Hunnicutt and Leffelman (2006), the goal of environmental change strategies is to create "health-enhancing environments" that include the following:

- *Economic environments* (i.e. financial costs and affordability)
- *Service environments* (i.e. accessibility to health care or patient education)
- *Social environments* (i.e. social support and peer pressure)
- *Cultural environments* (i.e. traditions of groups)
- *Psychological environments* (i.e. emotional learning environment)
- *Political environments* (i.e. support through policy change)
- *Built environments* (i.e. human-made surroundings for health-enhancing behaviors)

Planning environmental changes strategies requires the ability to think about macro environments within an ecological framework (see the Introduction to this book).

People who struggle with addiction tend to receive the bulk of addiction services when they are in the midst of crisis. Unfortunately, resources to help maintain sobriety once a person is stabilized are far more scarce. As a result, they may find themselves on a swinging pendulum – Rose referred to it as a "roller coaster of crisis and stability" throughout their lives. Straightening the stacks of brochures on a nearby counter, Rose continued to explain, "Never being on stable, solid ground is so hard on a person. It can impact relationships and opportunities for productivity. The Recovery Café program is here to provide a safe, steady space. It says to people, 'We'll be here for you. It's free, it's accessible. There will be people here to support you. It's a positive place for healing.'"

Services at the Recovery Café are intended to be "person-centered" and "meet a person where they are" in the process of recovery. The economic, service, social, cultural, psychological, political, and built environments at the Recovery Café are aimed to support health and constructive change.

As part of the organizational culture, each Recovery Café agrees to uphold specific core goals:

- Create a community space that is embracing and healing while being free of drug and alcohol use
- Nurture structures of loving accountability called recovery circles
- Empower every member to be a contributor
- Raise up "member leaders"
- Ensure responsible stewardship

Organizational culture refers to the "personality" of the organization (see Chapter 7). It is revealed through the norms, traditions, values, beliefs, and practices of an organization.

Golaszewski et al. (2008) states that organizational culture is related to "social standards of appropriate behavior." Organizational culture should permeate the system, encourage peer-support, and foster a sense of community.

Programs often reflect the culture of the organization that provides the programming, and program planners might find some resistance from organizations when the program seems contrary to the culture. In some cases, a new or revised program could be a catalyst for triggering positive changes to an organizational culture, should such change be needed.

The Café model differs from many other support services (e.g. recovery drop-in centers) because it requires a significant level of commitment from members. While there are no membership fees, members must commit to attending at least one recovery circle meeting per week and contribute in some way to the maintenance of the Café, such as helping to prepare meals or setting up/cleaning up the meeting spaces. Members must also be sober for 24-hours before attending a meeting. Members who show up under the influence of a substance can be a trigger for others, so they will be asked kindly by staff and member-leaders to return when they are at least 24-hours sober.

To punctuate the point, Rose smiled as she emphasized how membership reflects a type of contract between people at the Recovery Café. Membership governs the responsibilities and behaviors of the group members. Pulling out a colorful diagram from a nearby drawer, Rose highlighted the four components of Recovery Café participation:

1. Recovery Circles, led by a peer recovery coach, meet weekly for one hour to discuss personal recovery goals and report on success and challenges.
2. Sober social events, such as movie and game nights, allow members an opportunity to socialize in a drug- and alcohol-free space.
3. Education workshops of interest are offered to members and facilitated by volunteer subject experts from the community. These workshops are referred to as the Café School of Recovery, and topics might include journaling, yoga, relationship building, financial management, and restorative justice.
4. Lastly, community service is an aspect of the Recovery Café program where members use their time and talents to give back to the program in some way, such as helping to prepare meals or clean the meeting space.

"Each of these components require a lot of planning," Rose noted. "If we just try to throw an activity together at the last second, or send people out to do service without clear procedures and goals, things tend to backfire and our members lose confidence in us."

All Recovery Café activities emphasize the important role social support has proven to play in improving mental health, enhancing self-esteem, reducing loneliness, and promoting greater adherence to treatment plans. Members even seem to gain physical health and cardiovascular benefits. Rose has seen this again and again. She commented, "People change when they come here regularly. They have friends here who genuinely care about them, and that fundamentally changes how they take care of themselves."

Social support groups and activities are a part of many health promotion interventions because of their role in behavior change (see Zhao et al., 2022). People who come together to share experiences and support each other can be a powerful protector or buffer against stress.

- *Perceived social support* refers to the sense of belonging that people may develop among a group of people.
- *Received social support* refers to material benefits one person receives from another person or group.

Social networking is the act of looking for and developing relationships that can help people problem-solve, identify resources, or share information.

PROGRAM PLANNING STARTS WITH A VISION

The first Recovery Café was started in 2004 in Seattle, Washington, by a small group of community members who wanted to help their neighbors struggling with homelessness, addiction, and mental health issues. The effort was led by a woman named Killian Noe whose outreach work as a pastor led her to realize the dire need for recovery support services in her area. Killian's organizational skills and authentic capacity for connecting with others made her a natural leader for developing a program like Recovery Café. Though fierce in her advocacy for people in need, Killian is a slight woman with a warm, gentle voice. Those who meet her often remark that she exudes love and kindness and effortlessly brings out the best in others.

Wight et al. (2016) provides a six-step framework for planning a new health promotion program.

1. Define and understand the problem and its causes. Consider primary and secondary data to determine the risk factors for the health problem, as well as the context in which the problem occurs.
2. Clarify which causal or contextual factors are modifiable and have the greatest potential for change. Consider what potential changes would have the most effect and whether the program should focus on primary, secondary, or tertiary prevention. Consider what system (e.g. healthcare, education, criminal justice) the intervention would operate in, and if the system needs to be modified, as well.
3. Identify how to bring about change. Review intervention strategies known to be effective. Consider interventions that address multiple levels on the socio-ecological model (i.e. multiplicity) and that are supported by behavior change theory.
4. Determine how to deliver the change. Ensure that the necessary resources are secured for implementation.
5. Test and refine on a small scale. Consider if the intervention is an appropriate fit for the target population by conducting formative evaluations.
6. Collect sufficient evidence of effectiveness to justify continued implementation. Review that the intervention is working as intended, achieving desired objectives, and not inflicting harm or negative unintended effects.

The services provided by the first Recovery Café were much needed and so effective that membership in Seattle grew by the hundreds. By 2010, the Seattle Recovery Café had raised enough money to purchase their first building. Surrounding communities noted the program's growing success and wanted to replicate it. As a result, Recovery Café Network, a training and administrative support infrastructure, was launched in 2016 to assist nearby communities in their replication of the model. Since then, more than 25 Recovery Cafés have opened across North America. As satellite cafés have proliferated, each new Café must consider all the components needed to open and operate successfully, and to implement the Café with fidelity to the model.

When replicating a program, use checklists for the different components of the program and ensure each is being delivered according to the protocol. Carefully consider adapting the program components in ways that are culturally sensitive to the target population. Use evaluation tools to track outcomes.

Effective programs exhibit **cultural competency**, meaning that they "value diversity and ensure that activities, procedures, systems, and staffing are aligned to support the highest level of engagement and best outcomes for those who will participate" (Floersch, 2016). The following suggestions can foster cultural competence within programmatic efforts:

- Be aware of one's own biases (assess cultural assumptions)
- Address weaknesses in policies and procedures (reduce systematic biases toward certain groups)
- Be intentionally inclusive on planning team (include members from target populations who can inform the planning process)
- Define and understand the target population (identify who precisely is targeted and what characteristics are important to consider)
- Seek information from the target population (reflect their voices and views in the planning)
- Remember individuality (avoid stereotypes of groups, treat people as individuals)
- Continue learning (seek out information to assist with the steps above)

As part of local and peer-led efforts, each Recovery Café satellite has a different structure and tells a unique origin story molded by community needs and available resources. No Recovery Café looks the same as another, but all Cafés begin with a dedicated group of local people who endeavored to organize and promote the model as a form of substance use disorder intervention, with an emphasis on the recovery stage of the disorder. In some cases, a Recovery Café will form their own 501c3 nonprofit organization and lease a meeting space, or an established nonprofit organization with similar values can act as a fiscal sponsor and host site and run the Recovery Café as one of its programs.

> An intervention can be classified along an evidence-based continuum that indicates the extent to which evidence exists to support the use of an intervention (Puddy & Wilkins, 2011). The continuum is made up of the following ratings: *well-supported, supported, promising direction, emerging, undetermined, unsupported, and harmful*. These ratings are based on the rigor of the evaluations and the effectiveness in producing desired outcomes.
>
> The *Evidence-Based Practices Resource Center* (see Chapter 6) is a searchable depository of evidence-based mental health and substance abuse interventions. Other sources to identify research-based evidence on programs include the *Blueprints for Violence Prevention* (Blueprints, n.d.), *What Works Clearinghouse* (WWC, n.d.), the *Promising Practices Network for Children, Families, and Communities* (Rand, n.d.), among others.

In less than 20 years, the humble, local vision of Killian Noe and a small group of dedicated people has grown to a national organization supporting thousands of people in need. In 2019, the original Café held a fundraising campaign that raised $10 million dollars to support the continued efforts of the Recovery Café Network and the opening of Café satellites.

DEVELOPING, MAINTAINING, AND SUSTAINING A PROGRAM

Like Recovery Café Seattle, the local Recovery Café started with a small workgroup of dedicated volunteers who saw a need in their community. Community needs can be assessed in various ways. Initially, the process began with a listening tour through town to learn whether the community could benefit from and would support a Recovery Café. State epidemiological data had identified the town and the surrounding areas of the county as in dire need of recovery-based services based on high ranking for fatal opioid overdoses. However, although statistical data supported a need for recovery services in the area, Rose engaged in conversations with the community to learn whether they would actually participate in a service like Recovery Café.

While statistical data can point to a **normative need** for services – one supported by data – a **perceived need** is directed by the community, as they indicate what is desired and feasible in their current situation.

Despite a demonstrated statistical need, community members may lack trust in service providers or face other barriers to accessing services, such as isolation, lack of childcare, or fear of the unknown.

As part of the development process, the Recovery Café Network required the workgroup to submit a formal application, including a mission statement and a list of resources, skills, and life experiences that each workgroup member would bring to the effort.

Each workgroup member was also required to attend an intensive, online, multi-session training to learn more about the current policies and procedures for opening and operating a Recovery Café under the Seattle model. This training was delivered, in part, by Killian Noe and the other members of the original Seattle founding group. Overall, the training focused on implementation, which included officially learning about the technical operation of the Recovery Café program, identifying and moving into a physical brick and mortar location, hiring an executive director and café manager, recruiting board members, establishing a fiscal plan for sustainability of the café, and preparing for opening day.

Rose excitedly recounted the origin story of the local Recovery Café. The first step, she explained, was building community knowledge, enthusiasm, and support for the new Recovery Café, and motivating people to act and care about this issue.

It was really challenging, but in a fun way, to think about how to motivate business leaders, and faith leaders, and regular people to invest in the Recovery Café, either financially or with their time, social connections, or resources. We asked them about what creative ideas they had to help. Essentially, we were saying, 'Join us. We need you!'

To start, members of the workgroup had to identify and then reach out to leaders from various sectors – behavioral health centers, hospital outpatient programs, churches, neighborhood associations, criminal justice entities, county commissioners, city police, county law enforcement, emergency shelters, food banks, the university and community college, the local newspaper, and other groups like the rotary club. Rose reflected on the group's planning process, "It was important to learn who the biggest supporters of the effort would be, both in terms of who would open their pocketbooks to us, as well as who would spread the word, who would be willing to refer people to the Café, and who could contribute their talents to do social media outreach and logo design."

Community building is focused on assessing and then building upon the assets and capabilities of a community.

Asset-based Community Development (ABCD) is a process to catalog individual, community, and institutional capacities for positive action (Collaborative for Neighborhood Transformation, n.d.). In the ABCD approach, it is important to identify and mobilize existing but previously unrecognized assets to address needs.

Listening conversations, or one-on-one dialogue or small group conversations, are a critical part of ABCD because it is a way of discovering motivation, inviting participation, and developing relationships. Relationships build trust between individuals and across institutions.

Social capital is built through a network of relationships that exist within a community. Social capital is associated with trust among people and institutions who work together in collaborative action. Social capital increases the potential of a community to achieve change.

The workgroup also began to facilitate regular virtual informational meetings about the local Recovery Café where they would share information about the Café's philosophy and services, who might benefit, and how to refer a client or become a volunteer. Social media was instrumental in advertising these meetings where attendance varied from 1 to 8 attendees.

During the final training session with Killian Noe, the Recovery Café Network announced that they would provide each new Recovery Café satellite workgroup with $25,000 in seed money to help them to get started, along with another $25,000 in matching funds if the group could raise at least $10,000 on their own. Within the next year, the town's workgroup was able to raise the money through a weeklong social media campaign managed by a student intern from the local university.

FINDING A PHYSICAL LOCATION THAT MEETS PROGRAM NEEDS AND GOALS

The workgroup soon began to search for a physical site. Many Recovery Cafés begin in a small space that a larger, more established organization or nonprofit lends out to them. Or, in other situations, a fledgling Café might pay an organization a small fee for renting the space until they can raise money to purchase property of their own.

The workgroup reached out to several like-minded organizations that might be interested in housing a Café, but each organization had limitations related to the layout and capacity of the available space or its availability. Most Cafés, by design, are open during weekends and mealtimes but such times were also popular for other organizations, meaning they were unlikely to have extra space to lend out.

Another challenge was ensuring that the location of the local Recovery Café would be inviting and avoid being an emotional trigger for people who might want to access it. For example, one location option was in a building that used to be the county jail.

Rose said, "We didn't want potential members to feel intimidated by the location of the Café. Some people in recovery have a criminal history, and we didn't want to re-traumatize them with a reminder of that trauma."

The Café location also needed to have a kitchen, dining area, and ample meeting space, for both small and large groups, so the location needed to be welcoming, nonjudgmental, centrally located, safe, and accessible by public transportation.

"In some ways," Rose recalled, "it felt like we were searching for a needle in a haystack."

Eventually, the group found a location in the heart of Downtown nestled in a building that used to be a department store. The building ran adjacent to the public bus line and had free and ample parking. The owners of the building, a nondenominational church, occupied part of the facility and had made it their mission to lease out unused space for a discounted rate to nonprofit organizations.

The workgroup acknowledged that it was not ideal for a Recovery Café to share space with a church, as some members might have experienced religious trauma and might avoid settings with a religious affiliation. However, the building was quite spacious and had multiple entrances so that those who entered the Café may not even realize it was sharing space with a church. As the church only occupied a small portion of the building, the Café would be in a separate wing to indicate that it was not a program within the church. The workgroup also felt that the nondenominational and open and affirming nature of the church aligned in more ways than not with Recovery Café values.

Recovery Café welcomes individuals regardless of race/ethnicity, gender identity, sexuality, nationality, and creed. Many substance recovery groups in the United States, and particularly in rural areas, are **faith-based**, meaning that are affiliated with Christianity or a general belief in a higher power. **Alcoholics Anonymous**, for example, established in 1935 and commonly known as AA, includes a 12-step program where Step 2 is "belief that a Power greater than ourselves can restore us to sanity." Though AA is a popular recovery pathway worldwide, with an estimation of over two million members, many people in recovery chose a different pathway.

Recovery Café welcomes individuals regardless of their pathway – whether they participate in therapeutic recovery, medication-assisted treatment, or opt for an independent solo recovery.

The space available to the Café included a kitchen, large meeting room, and several smaller rooms that could be used for storage, staff offices, and private meetings spaces. The Café workgroup was given permission to put up signage and paint the walls in a color palette that was warm, inviting, and consistent with their branding.

After one full month of preparing the site, the Recovery Café quietly launched a **soft opening**, inviting a limited audience to experience the space and provide feedback about layout and logistics. The Café's **grand opening** occurred weeks later and was marked by a festive event hosted at the Café and attended by the mayor, a journalist from the local newspaper, and several other key figures in the community.

The first day of a program is often called the **program launch, program rollout**, or **program kickoff**. Program planners can consider launching a program on a date that coincides with another traditionally well-attended event that might help promote the program, such as hosting the launch on the weekend of a county fair or parade.

Ways to promote a new program include contests, games, meals, ribbon cuttings, or appearances by well-known individuals, such as elected officials, CEOs, or other people affected by the problem. Program planning can solicit news coverage of the launch by contacting the press and providing them with a **press release** that includes newsworthy data or information related to the problem and how the program will help address it.

A year later, the Recovery Café was bustling with activity. At noon on a Wednesday, a member-leader named Walter was confidently leading group affirmations before lunch was served. Though he could not stand erect to his full height and leaned a portion of his body weight on a cane, Walter energetically commanded the attention of the room as he called upon those who had taken a seat in the dining area to share something they felt positive about in that moment. More than 25 people were seated in the space and nearly everyone opted to share their thoughts. The tone of the room was upbeat, lighthearted, and connected.

Next, Walter reminded the group of who signed up for clean-up chores that day, delivered a few announcements about upcoming activities, and led them through five minutes of silence, a well-established ritual at the Café. As they settled into silence, the dining room filled with the pleasant odor of warm food floating in from the adjacent kitchen.

In the year since its grand opening, the Recovery Café was its own independent 501c3 organization. The budget had expanded, thanks to a fundraising breakfast and auction event, as well as significant, external grant funding. A Board of Directors had been established, and Rose was increasingly comfortable and confident in her role as Executive Director. A lively, attentive young woman who had recently graduated from college had been hired as the Café Manager. Social work student interns continued to cycle in and out and some chose to continue to volunteer as Café Companions. As part of the peer-led nature of the program and based in the principle of reciprocity, or giving back, nearly a dozen members had been promoted to member-leader status and led Circles and other programming as part of their Café membership. Café hours had expanded to four days a week from 11 a.m. to 3 p.m.

So much had happened in a seemingly small amount of time, and all had begun with a small group of committed people who believed they had the power to change someone's world.

DISCUSSION QUESTIONS

1. What benefits come from the approach of "everyone is in recovery from something"? How might this attitude help people seeking recovery from substance use disorders?

2. How have you seen the power of connection benefit you or others? What prevents connection from happening? How can we, as a community, make connection a more natural occurrence?

3. Consider the challenges to radical hospitality that might arise when managing a program like the Recovery Café. What sort of program policies may need to be implemented to ensure that members are following the rules and contributing to the safety of the program?

4. What are some advantages and disadvantages of requiring certain things of members before they are allowed to participate in a program? What do you think about the requirements of the Recovery Café?

5. Brainstorm examples of unhealthy coping habits related to sensation, approval, control, shame, blame, and self-loathing. How might it be difficult to break these habits?

6. How can program planners incorporate environmental change strategies into their planning? Which environments might be most difficult to account for? Explain.

7. What is the difference between perceived social support and received social support? Why does this difference matter? How can they become the same thing?

8. How have social support activities been integrated into health interventions you have been a part of? What did the social support activities consist of? In your experience, how does social support help motivate behavior change?

9. What can go wrong when programs are not culturally competent?

10. Why might it be justified to adopt a program lower on the evidence-based continuum? What are the risks of doing so?

11. What helps you become interested in a community event or service? What attempts have you seen to publicize an event or service that failed to get you interested?

ACTIVITIES

1. Watch Johann Hari's TED Talk (2015) listed in the references below and explore Bruce Alexander's extensive body of work (www.brucekalexander.com). What do you think about the rat experiment? How might it apply to human behavior?

2. Refer to the six-step framework when planning a new health promotion program. Review the chapter to find examples of each of these steps regarding the creation or adoption of the Recovery Café program. What steps appear to be absent or unclear? What could have been done differently regarding these steps?

3. Refer to the six-step framework when planning a new health promotion program. Using these steps, describe how you would plan the development and implementation of a new program, such as an after-school program to help prevent teen drug use or a program that educates members of the community about an environmental hazard.

REFERENCES

Blueprints (n.d.). Center for the Study and Prevention of Violence. https://www.blueprintsprograms.org/

Collaborative for Neighborhood Transformation (n.d.). ABCD Toolkit. https://resources.depaul.edu/abcd-institute/resources/Documents/WhatisAssetBasedCommunity Development.pdf

Floersch, B. (2016). *Planning Culturally Competent Programs*. The Grantsmanship Center. https://www.tgci.com/blog/2016/06/planning-culturally-competent-programs

Golaszewski, T., Allen, J., & Edington, D. (2008). Working together to create supportive environments in worksite health promotion. *American Journal of Health Promotion: AJHP*, *22*(4), 1–10, iii. https://doi.org/10.4278/0890-1171-22.5.TAHP-1

Hari, J. (2015). *Chasing the scream: The first and last days of the war on drugs*. New York: Bloomsbury.

Hunnicutt, D. & Leffelman, B. (2006). WELCOAs 7 benchmarks of success. *Absolute Advantage*, *6*(1), 2–29.

Puddy, R. W. & Wilkins, N. (2011). *Understanding Evidence Part 1: Best Available Research Evidence. A Guide to the Continuum of Evidence of Effectiveness*. Centers for Disease Control and Prevention. https://www.cdc.gov/violenceprevention/pdf/understanding_evidence-a.pdf

Rand (n.d.). *Promising Practices*. https://www.rand.org/well-being/social-and-behavioral-policy/projects/promising-practices.html

Recovery Café Network (2017, April 3). *Home – Recovery Café Network*. https://recoverycafenetwork.org/

TED (2015, July 9). *Everything You Think You Know About Addiction is Wrong* | Johann Hari [Video]. YouTube. https://www.youtube.com/watch?v=PY9DcIMGxMs

Wight, D., Wimbush, E., Jepson, R., & Doi, L. (2016). Six steps in quality intervention development (6SQuID). *Journal of Epidemiology and Community Health*, *70*(5), 520–525. https://doi.org/10.1136/jech-2015-205952

What Works Clearinghouse, WWC. (n.d.). Ies.ed.gov. https://ies.ed.gov/ncee/wwc

Zhao, X., Jin, A., & Hu, B. (2022). How do perceived social support and community social network alleviate psychological distress during COVID-19 lockdown? The mediating role of residents' epidemic prevention capability. *Frontiers in Public Health*, *10*, 763490. https://doi.org/10.3389/fpubh.2022.763490

CHAPTER

10

GRASSROOTS COMMUNITY ORGANIZING

ASSESSING READINESS FOR CHANGE

In this chapter, we highlight the story of Jeannette and Craig on their respective journeys in community organizing. In program planning, community organizing is an intervention strategy that can pay huge dividends for the community as large-scale investments can be made in public health.

After implementing a successful symposium on substance use disorders (see Chapter 8), Jeannette O'Augusta, a university professor, considered whether the community was truly ready to launch an addictions coalition that could ensure the symposium event was not a "one and done" project. Jeannette had a bright personality, long curly hair,

Health Promotion Planning: Learning from the Accounts of Public Health Practitioners,
First Edition. Jean Marie S. Place, Jonel Thaller, and Scott S. Hall.
© 2024 John Wiley & Sons, Inc. Published 2024 by John Wiley & Sons, Inc.

and was optimistic by nature. She was eager to get more involved in her community, beyond the ivory tower of her academic institution. She and her fellow planning committee members wanted their actions to have a larger impact on prevention, treatment, and recovery services in their area, but they needed the help of local professionals and the lay public. Most symposium attendees had indicated an interest in participating in a community coalition, but coalition building does not happen on its own, and everyone would need to be willing and able to put in the work.

The Community Readiness Model (CRM) is a useful tool that encourages stakeholders to review their community's readiness for change in five different dimensions:

- Community knowledge of efforts
- Leadership
- Community climate
- Community knowledge of the issue
- Resources

According to this model, community readiness includes the following stages:

- *Absence of awareness* – the community does not recognize the health issue.
- *Denial or resistance* – there is little recognition or concern among community members about the health issue.
- *Vague awareness* – the community may be concerned about the health issue, but the motivation to address it is low.
- *Preplanning* – the community recognizes that action is needed, but there is a lack of focused activity around the health issue.
- *Preparation* – leaders in the community begin to plan and support approaches to addressing the health issue.
- *Initiation* – the community begins activities to address the health issue.
- *Stabilization* – the community activities are supported by administrators and other community leaders.
- *Confirmation/expansion* – activities have been implemented and the community is comfortable with addressing the health issue.

- *High level of community ownership* – data are being gathered that support the efforts, and the approach may be replicated in other communities. (Rural health Information Hub, n.d.).

The community's stage of change depends on a community's attitudes, knowledge, efforts, and resources. Once the community's stage of readiness has been determined, there are strategies for moving forward toward greater programmatic success and sustainability.

Trained in public health practices and program planning, Jeannette referred to the Community Readiness Model (CRM) to consider where her community might fall in terms of readiness to build a coalition to address addiction. Jeannette recognized that most members of the community already had an awareness of substance use problems, which is the first stage in the CRM. Unfortunately, their county was ranked high in the state for overdose deaths, and the local newspaper often headlined stories about drugs: fathers with felonies, mothers charged with neglect, deaths due to drunk driving. Addressing addiction was an issue that came up in Q&A sessions with city council and mayoral candidates, and many people indicated they knew someone with substance use disorder, often within their own family.

Likewise, Jeannette did not think her community was in the "denial" phase, which is characterized by the feeling that nothing can be done to stop the problem. Support groups existed in the community and many churches had added recovery-oriented ministries to support their congregations. It is true, however, that there was substantial miscommunication and incorrect knowledge about drug use, with plenty of social media posts offering stigmatized opinions about people who use drugs and insisting that quitting cold turkey was the only way to sobriety.

Vague awareness was the stage that resonated with Jeannette the most when considering the community's relationship to the growing substance misuse issue. In this phase, there is acknowledgement that the problem exists, but no leadership has stepped up to tackle it.

It is important to know how willing and prepared a community is to take action. It is unwise to push for change beyond what a community is ready to take on because of the high likelihood of failure. Even communities that are high in resources can fail at an effort if they are low in readiness. Understanding a community's stage of readiness helps to determine where change agents should start in their efforts to address a problem.

Jeannette felt pulled to act, but she was unsure of where to start. She felt passionate about the issue based on data she had seen and stories she had read, but recognized herself as an outsider to the part of the community that was affected most by substance use disorder. She recalled, "I had never actually had an addiction problem, and, I'm embarrassed to admit it, but I didn't know anyone with a substance use disorder either, at least not that I knew of."

Although Jeannette was willing to take on the role as an initial coalition organizer, she knew her limitations as a credible leader given her lack of personal experience. She lived in a well-maintained and somewhat insulated neighborhood just a few blocks away from the university campus where she worked and miles away from the parts of the city most affected by poverty, homelessness, and the gravest effects of substance misuse. She had heard of students who drank too much at fraternity parties, and she knew there was great concern about students drinking and driving. However, when she walked out of her home, she did not come across used needles on her lawn or see people living in tents because addiction had zapped their ability to maintain a job. Still, as a researcher and faculty member at the local university, Jeannette was trained to look at data and interpret trends, and she clearly recognized the profound challenges with substance misuse in her community and wanted to contribute to the betterment of the whole community.

JOINING FORCES WITH LOCAL LEADERS

While Jeannette was exploring what a coalition could look like and whom to invite as co-organizers, she met a man named Craig Boullion, who was known as a street pastor in one of the hardest hit neighborhoods in town. Having lived in this neighborhood his entire life, Craig was recognized by the community as an insider. He was known for helping people who lived with substance use disorder, especially those who were unhoused and living on the street. He had started to welcome neighbors into the garage adjacent to his home to strategize a plan of action. By organizing these informal meetings, Craig had taken initiative to enact change from within the troubled community. Craig's efforts were grassroots, or a bottom-up initiative, and when Jeannette and Craig started working together, they formed a powerful team.

By herself, Jeannette did not know enough about the impacted community in the southside of the city to be helpful, but Craig did. As a lifelong neighborhood resident, he had already gained entry and established credibility in the community. He had spent decades visiting folks on their front porches, eating meals with them, spontaneously helping kids with homework or other tasks, and shooting hoops with teenagers outside his back door.

Jeannette had crossed paths with Craig at several community meetings, and they had become fast friends as they spent time together talking about issues related to substance use. Craig sensed that Jeannette was sincere in her effort to help and was eager to inform her about the problems his neighbors faced in getting access to resources.

Jeannette recalled, "Craig was the real deal. He had a calling to help his neighbors, and they saw that and trusted him. In this way, he was also a gatekeeper. There was no way for me to do work in his neighborhood without his trust and blessing." She continued, "Craig took me around the neighborhood on multiple occasions, introducing me to people as his 'friend,' and letting them know I was willing to help. He invited me in to do the work he had already been doing for years." Craig was trusted and well-respected in his community, and with time and his stamp of approval, people came to respect Jeannette, too.

Gatekeeper is a term that implies one must pass through a particular entryway to gain access to people on the other side (Wright, 1994). Gatekeepers know the power dynamics of their community, how it functions, and how to appropriately accomplish change within it.

Gatekeepers generally understand the culture of a community. It is important to work toward cultural competence and practice cultural sensitivity. One must be humble and understand that one is not the expert on the community and should rely on insiders' knowledge.

STRENGTHENING RELATIONSHIPS THROUGH GRASSROOTS ORGANIZING

Craig eventually invited Jeannette to join the Sunday evening gatherings held in his garage. She recalled colorful Christmas lights hanging from the beams of the garage, a dozen or so people sitting in lawn chairs, crowded around mowers, bikes, and garden supplies.

Craig and his neighbors had come together to discuss the problems substance misuse was causing in their neighborhood. People were dying from overdose and many neighbors knew the people being wheeled out of homes on stretchers. The group was established because they wanted to organize and do something to tackle the growing concern. Craig became the de-facto leader, partly because it was his garage, and partly because of his leadership skills.

Though Craig had grown up in this neighborhood, he had left for a short time to pursue a college education before returning to the familiar streets of the neighborhood. Recently, he had taken a six-week online course on community organizing from the Harvard School of Public Health, but he did not present himself as an elite or an expert.

"I may have gone to Harvard," he joked, referring to his online course. "But I'm just like anyone else around here. When I hold these meetings, I'm just here to facilitate. We've taken votes on every decision that was made, and I definitely didn't stand out in front of everyone and tell them what to do."

Effective community organizers typically possess a specific set of skills that make them good at what they do (Mondros & Wilson, 1994).

- First, they are visionaries who can see beyond a problem and visualize a potential change in outcomes. They are driven by this image and are willing to put in the work to make it happen.
- Second, they thoroughly understand the problem, appropriately assess strengths and challenges, develop strategies to mitigate obstacles, and communicate effectively about plans.
- Third, they are skilled at building structures that can retain volunteers and are proficient at organizational management like overseeing task groups and raising money.
- Fourth, they have superior communication and relational skills that keep everyone motivated and moving forward toward a goal.

As part of establishing a presence in the larger community, Craig and the group of neighbors wanted a name with which to brand themselves. They came up with several creative suggestions, and the group voted on the name *Southside Pride*. As they discussed the variety of issues present in the neighborhood, namely related to addiction and mental illness, they recognized the need to establish group guidelines for their community meetings. Craig led them through an exercise he learned from his online public health course, and the group developed these rules:

1. Personal things shared within this group stay in the group.
2. No judgment because of our struggles.
3. Everyone is included regardless of race, age, religion, gender, etc.

4. When someone is speaking, we will respect by listening.
5. We will not interrupt each other.
6. Everyone has an equal voice in discussions.
7. We will make decisions by consensus.

The group also formalized a mission statement for what they wanted to accomplish: "Southside Pride is focused on bringing addiction services to the southside. Southside Pride aims to facilitate justice by urgently bringing inclusive mental health and addiction services to southside residents."

As the group gained more purpose and function, it began to act as a **taskforce**, convening for a specific purpose and timeframe. But unlike a taskforce set up by another body or committee, they organized themselves in a "grassroots" manner.

Craig joked, "I think other people in town thought that Southside Pride was this huge group of people, like 200 or more of us." He laughed, "That totally wasn't the case. We were only 15 or so strong, but we had an impact, and people were listening to us."

Jeannette recalls that some neighbors showed up every Sunday night, and there was always food available, which partially fueled steady attendance. This same group also showed up on Thursday nights for the weekly church meal in their neighborhood. They developed a Facebook page for Southside Pride and created an infographic to depict what they wanted to see happen. Jeannette was an active participant in the group. She looked forward to these Sunday meetings and eagerly took a seat in Craig's garage to engage in discussions about what should be done.

Community groups tend to be comprised of people with different activity levels and contributions. **Active participants** take part in most activities. **Occasional participants** may show up to meetings irregularly. **Supporting participants** support activities in nonactive ways by speaking positively about the group, referring others to it, or donating financially.

Programs fueled by community groups benefit from a variety of contributions, but should ensure that enough active participants are involved to carry out the work necessary for a program to progress.

BUILDING CONSENSUS AND WORKING TOGETHER

As an affiliate of the local university and someone trained in public health and community change strategies, Jeannette had important information to add to group discussions. She brought data to the meeting, integrating facts and figures into the anecdotes that others shared.

"I felt that sharing some state-wide data and research on substance use disorder would help us better interpret our observations and communicate with others how these statistics manifest in real life. Sometimes you can be stuck in the data and forget that real people are involved. Other times, you can be so close to the problem that you forget important cultural, institutional, and contextual factors that contribute to it," Jeanette explained.

The group seemed to appreciate Jeannette's data sharing, seeing it as an important step in the process of assessment, prior to determining goals and priorities to focus on. Craig, perhaps intuitively, seemed to have a knack for seeing the bigger picture. In one meeting, Craig recalled with some frustration, that some members were sharing derogatory stories about others in the neighborhood, particularly those who were selling drugs.

While drug dealers existed in the neighborhood and many neighbors worried about the harm they caused, Craig kept asking the question *why*. "Why were they selling drugs? Why did they need money? Why weren't they in school or have productive employment?" He said, "We kept going until we reached the root reason. The ultimate answer was that people struggled to have enough to survive. The deepest answer was isolation." Craig maintained that this process of moving beyond stigmatized views of others was critical for group cohesion and a larger-than-self commitment to the cause.

United in their desire for a healthier community, the group was ready to determine their main request of city leaders who had the resources to help their struggling neighborhood. Post-pandemic, the city would be receiving federal funding as part of the American Rescue Plan (ARP). The group hoped to effectively direct the incoming funding toward their identified concerns, helping to make a real impact for their neighbors, family members, and friends.

One of the community's major problems, according to Southside Pride members, was the fact that many of their neighbors who were experiencing behavioral health problems had no place to go other than the emergency room or jail. Craig said, "People talking to themselves and walking the streets didn't belong in either of those places, but there was nowhere else to take them to get help." The group wondered if the hospital network could be leveraged to address the crisis they were seeing on their streets. The local hospital network with an asset in the community, especially because it had a robust behavioral health workforce.

After these energetic discussions, it was time to decide specifically what the group wanted to accomplish. Craig led the group to vote on every decision. Part of the reason for this, according to Craig, was that many group members had never been involved with a taskforce before and were unaccustomed to giving feedback. Voting was a structured way to gain consensus and move forward.

The group voted to advocate for a 24/7 behavioral health crisis center to be located on the southside of the city. This could be used by law enforcement as an alternative outcome to taking people to jail. The center would be a 24-hour drop-in center for people in crisis with mental or behavioral health problems, like substance use disorders. Guests would be able to detox at the center safely and receive case management for housing, treatment, and other concerns. The vote was 100% in favor of moving this proposal forward. Craig recognized that getting everyone on board is not always that easy. In this case, though, he said, "the need was obvious."

The Centers for Disease Control (CDC) suggests that building consensus is a useful way to establish a group's priorities. However, finding consensus can be hard to do! The CDC provides several suggestions:

- Try to avoid the thinking that there is only one way to achieve a goal. Instead, remember that there may be multiple pathways to a solution.

- Do not limit healthy conflict when deciding upon the goals and priorities of a group because conflict can lead to solutions that incorporate multiple perspectives, especially when participants are committed to listening and communicating respectfully.

COLLABORATING ACROSS INSTITUTIONAL BOUNDARIES

The group felt some relief having come to a consensus on their end goal. Yet, there was still much work to do to convince stakeholders, such as elected officials, nonprofit leaders, hospital administrators, and other community development specialists, to support the plan. Craig described several strategies to introduce stakeholders to the idea of a 24/7 crisis center and to get people to unite around this idea.

The group organized an in-person rally at a park where he called on the county commissioners to verbally issue their support for a crisis center. On another day, the group requested the use of a church van and drove half a dozen people, including the sheriff, city council members, a judge, and the deputy mayor, to an established crisis center in another city. They toured the facility and asked questions about implementation. Craig recalled, "Little by little, they were beginning to see how the crisis center idea could become a reality in our town." Two more tours to crisis centers across the state were organized. As part of the last tour, Craig planned to ask people in positions of power to verbally commit to use their organizational resources to support a crisis center in the southside of the city.

Craig was very pleased with what happened next. Dr. Snow, the director of a major medical group in town and a fierce advocate for people with substance use disorders, testified to the importance of crisis centers as a waystation on the road to recovery, which became instrumental to convincing other stakeholders to support the cause.

Craig leaned back in his chair as he remembered the enthusiasm around this time. "We were doing it together. There was just so much momentum." Jeannette jumped in – an apparent fact checker – and added that some groups were more difficult to get on board than others. For example, a local homeless shelter had been reticent to support the crisis center because of past experiences that had resulted in legal action. A mental health network lacked the trust of the community to take a leading role in the crisis center project, although they were the designated community behavioral health center. Jeannette recalled a conference call where some stakeholders blamed other organizations for gaps in services. She remembered, "There were many phone calls and meetings with stakeholders to try to answer all the various concerns they had. We tried to make people see the cross-cutting benefits to the proposed crisis center, even though people had various, diverging interests."

Sometimes agencies with similar goals engage in so-called "**turf battles**." These are especially likely to occur when groups are competing for limited resources, as is typically the case for health-related programs. For example, agencies within the same community that sponsor substance use disorder initiatives can feel threatened by a new program with similar objectives. Will this new program draw attention away from the existing programs? Will grant funders and donors use their money to support the new program instead? Will the new program do things the "right" way? Turf battles can hinder efforts to deliver effective programs.

Scholars at the Harvard Law School offer three strategies for avoiding turf battles (Shonk, 2020):

1. Focus on a shared goal or identity. Thinking about the long-term outcomes that organizations are working toward can help unite them in working together instead of feeling in competition with one another. Letting the goal drive their efforts more than organizational pride or relevancy can help agencies keep in mind what matters most and work together for that purpose.

2. Distinguish between sacred issues and pseudo-sacred issues. Sacred issues – those that are off limits to negotiation on moral or philosophical grounds – might actually be negotiable under certain conditions. In such cases, these issues can be labeled as *pseudo-sacred*. For example, an agency might dig its heels in against supporting efforts that seem to enable more substance use among people in recovery (e.g. using certain medications that counter the effects of withdrawal symptoms), but after learning more about how such techniques have been used to save lives of adolescents, agree to explore the possibility of a program that uses such intervention at high schools. As agencies try to collaborate while sharing the same turf, each needs to be clear on what is truly nonnegotiable and be slower to instantly dismiss diverse perspectives.

3. *Gradual Reduction of Tension, or GRIT.* Hostility between organizations can be reduced through genuine communication and building trust. Learning of each other's hopes and experiences can help overcome mistrust. Making small concessions to one another displays sincere desires to get along. Avoid escalating conflict by responding peacefully.

Program planners should be aware of the potential for turf battles and work to minimize them. An important component of developing programming is to know what programming is already offered. Choosing to collaboratively build off what is already being done can be more effective than creating a new program.

Many questions arose throughout the refinement process of the crisis center proposal, but a turning point occurred when the hospital network agreed to host meetings and create sub-committees to explore various dimensions of the project, including facility/location needs, funding, communication, services, staffing, and transport.

Still, Craig set his coffee cup down on the round café table as he discussed what he perceived as an error in the make-up of the eventual subcommittees organized by the hospital leaders. "Neighbors of the southside should have been invited to participate in the subcommittees and provide input. It was their idea to advocate for a crisis center, and they were pushed out when more powerful stakeholders moved into the discussions." Although Craig recognized that subcommittees were organized and coordinated by the hospital network to discuss detail-oriented planning, he resisted the idea that neighbors would not be able to contribute. "We have to remember to bring in the voices of the people affected by the problem. If not, programs are created that don't truly address their needs."

Subcommittees can complete tasks that contribute to the larger goal. These and other questions may be relevant to the work of program planning, depending on the project:

Facility/Location

- Where should the facility or program be located? In what area? In an existing building?
- How large of a facility will be needed?
- What amenities need to be available?
- What should the hours of the facility or program be?

Funding

- What grants are secured?
- What grants are available?
- How will this facility or program be funded as initial grants become exhausted?
- What will the budget look like for this endeavor?

Communication Needs

- How will information (e.g. phone numbers, facility services) be communicated to the public?
- How will education be given to providers and others who encounter clients?
- How will community stakeholders be kept informed of project updates?

Services

- How should services at the facility be aligned with those available in the community?
- How should referral channels be built?
- What are the services that will be offered on-site at the facility?

Staffing

- What are the required qualifications from staff?
- How many full-time employees will be required to fulfill services?
- What types of staff training should be required?
- How do we leverage volunteers?

Transport

- Who should make up the transport team retrieving the client?
- How far will the transport service be offered? What is the scope of services?
- What types of resources are needed to make the scope of services possible?
- What groups will physically transport the clients both to and from the facility?

FUNDING THE PROJECT

The community's ARP funds needed to be used to address mental health and addiction concerns in communities, but entities vying for the funds had to make a case for them. "It was the perfect opportunity to advocate for the crisis center," Craig said.

The President of City Council called Craig to invite members of Southside Pride to present at a City Council meeting on the crisis center proposal, and Craig described how he prepared his neighbors to provide testimony at the City Council meeting. He gathered stories dictated to him from his neighbors who were suffering food insecurity, mental illness, and a myriad of unsuccessful attempts at treatment in the convoluted mental health treatment system. All the group members had struggled to access services at some point. As Craig condensed their stories into talking points, he coached them on ending their declarations as follows: "And that is why I'm advocating for a 24-hour crisis center for mental health and addiction."

On the day of the City Council meeting, the room was full of neighbors from the southside, about 50 in total. One neighbor's hands visibly shook as she stood and shared her story. She ended her testimony with a powerful plea: "We have to have a safe place where people can show up." Members of the audience clapped vigorously as they gave her a standing ovation. ARP funding was approved to support the crisis center.

As is often the case, additional funding was needed to enhance and sustain the program over time, resulting in the group actively searching for more funding sources. When a state-level grant opportunity was released, the stakeholders kicked into action to write a proposal to supplement ARP funds and provide enough monies for the renovation of a physical space as well as the first two years of operation for the crisis center. It would take constant effort to ensure the crisis center had the resources to fully function, but to the members of Southside Pride, the effort meant that lives were changing in their community.

Grant opportunities are typically announced to the public with very specific guidelines for application. Governments and private and public foundations fund what is important to them and that aligns with their mission. Thus, grant-seekers must be clear about how their particular program will help advance the goals of the funder.

Organizations seeking grants must meet the requirements for eligibility (e.g. be a not-for-profit agency located in a certain area) to receive the funding, but even eligible programs have their funding proposals rejected because the demand for funding is typically much greater than what is available. Grant-seeking can be very competitive and proposals should be written with great care and should clearly and completely address all the requirements for any given proposal. There is no universal template for grant proposals – each can have its own instructions.

Grants differ in their purposes and application. Common types of grants available to nonprofit organizations include the following (Hoy, 2022):

1. **Seed money** or **start-up grants** are used for helping an organization get established. Usually, this money is awarded with the understanding that the agency will seek additional funding elsewhere to sustain the organization.

2. **Project grants** fund specific programs provided by an existing organization. Money must be spent on things related to achieving the goals of the project.

3. **Capacity building grants** provide funds that can be added to existing resources and efforts to increase the capacity or capability of the organization to provide its services. The focus tends to be on increasing or improving organizational processes rather than on a single project of program.

4. **Operating fund grants** assist with monthly expenses associated with running the organization.

5. **Research grants**, in the case of an organization, support research that provides critical data for the organization, such as a community-wide needs assessment or the outcome evaluation of a program.

6. **Endowment grants** come from nonprofits who have endowments that earn interest, and funders might contribute to such endowments to incentivize successful programming.

7. **Facilities and equipment grants**, also known as **capital grants**, support the physical space and equipment needs of an organization so it can focus its resources on its programming.

8. **Technical assistance grants** are used to hire experts or consultants who can assist with specific tasks outside the abilities of an organization's staff but are needed to run an organization (e.g. marketing, technology, accounting).

9. **Conditional grants** require that certain criteria must be met before the funding is awarded. For example, once an organization fundraises a certain amount of money, a matching amount will then be awarded by the funder.

10. **In-kind grants** are often provided instead of awarding money. Other types of resources are granted, such as a vehicle, computer equipment, office supplies, or meal catering for program participants.

For Jeannette and Craig, the taskforce they had convened for a short, time-limited time had been successful. A **coalition** – a formal alliance between organizations, individuals, and groups that dedicates itself to advocating on an issue – was just beginning. They imagined together a bright future where a budding coalition of community members would plan and implement programs for substance use prevention, treatment, and recovery.

DISCUSSION QUESTIONS

1. How could you go about determining the level of community readiness for a certain program? What would be the biggest challenges in doing so?

2. What are the benefits that both insiders and outsiders bring to addressing a community problem?

3. Why might an outsider experience some pushback from those within a community? What kind of pushback might Jeannette have received if she had not worked with Craig?

4. What are the advantages and disadvantages of building off of an established program compared to creating a new program?

5. Why might grassroots efforts to begin a community program be particularly successful? Why might they particularly struggle?

6. When trying to build consensus, what is the difference between "healthy conflict" and conflict that is more problematic?

7. What human tendencies do we have that can contribute to engaging in turf battles?

8. How can program planners prepare to successfully make use of subcommittees? Where does planning fit in?

ACTIVITIES

1. Imagine you feel the need to "do something" about a problem in your community that you care about. Identify the problem and then look online for an existing program that addresses this problem. Describe how you might be able to collaborate with the agency offering the program to build off of or expand the program. Describe what you see would be potential causes of turf battles and what you would do to minimize them.

2. Refer to the 10 types of grants commonly available to nonprofit organizations. Look online for an example of at least five of these grant types. Document what is required by the funder in each case to qualify for the grant, what the grant can fund, and how much money is available for each grant proposal. Describe what you learned from this experience.

REFERENCES

Hoy, T. (2022, June 28). *10 Types of Nonprofit Grants: Does Your Organization Qualify for Funding?* BoardEffect. https://www.boardeffect.com/blog/types-of-nonprofit-grants/

Mondros, J. B. & Wilson, S. M. (1994). *Organizing for Power and Empowerment.* Columbia Press.

Rural Health Information Hub (n.d.). Community Readiness Model. https://www.ruralhealthinfo.org/toolkits/health-promotion/2/program-models/community-readiness

Shonk, K. (2020). *In Group Negotiation, Avoid Turf Battle.* Program on Negotiation. Harvard Law School. https://www.pon.harvard.edu/daily/business-negotiations/group-negotiation-avoid-turf-battle/

Wright, P. A. (1994). *Technical Assistance Bulletin: A Key Step in Developing Prevention Materials is to Obtain Expert and Gatekeepers' Reviews.* CSAP Communications Team.

CHAPTER

TRAUMA-INFORMED CARE

CREATING HEALTH COMMUNICATION CAMPAIGNS FOR PUBLIC AWARENESS

This chapter illustrates how grant funding was used to implement a county change team to raise awareness about a particular approach to substance misuse intervention – trauma-informed care. A formalized needs assessment helped the team determine strategies for delivering their message.

Health Promotion Planning: Learning from the Accounts of Public Health Practitioners,
First Edition. Jean Marie S. Place, Jonel Thaller, and Scott S. Hall.
© 2024 John Wiley & Sons, Inc. Published 2024 by John Wiley & Sons, Inc.

At the monthly Chamber of Commerce networking breakfast, Wendy Radcliff, a professor at the local university, and her graduate assistant Mae sighed with relief as they approached the informational table reserved by their team and set down the large load they were carrying. They had just moved several boxes full of tabling supplies and swag – a customized tablecloth, multiple signage, color-printed flyers and pamphlets, stickers, buttons, T-shirts, candy, and a jar to collect business cards – from Wendy's parked car and into the ballroom of the convention center. Their load was not particularly heavy, but it was cumbersome. One of the signs was an A-frame style with their organization's logo and contact info printed on both sides and intended to stand 4 ft tall when placed on the ground.

Both Wendy and Mae were dressed in matching black T-shirts with white lettering. Their shirts read "Is your _____ trauma-informed?" meant to inspire reflection on whether you are engaging in trauma-informed care in whatever spaces you occupy. On the back of the shirts were listed five common principles of trauma-informed care:

- Safety
- Choice
- Collaboration
- Trustworthiness
- Empowerment

Colorful stickers encased in one of the boxes, 150 of them in total, also included the question "Is your _____ trauma-informed?" along with a QR code leading to more information about trauma-informed care. The public could fill in the blank: *Is your healthcare provider trauma-informed? your therapist? pharmacist? bank teller? bus driver?*

Wendy kept her fingers crossed that people who read their T-shirts and the stickers would understand what the question meant. When her team came up with the interrogative phrase and voted unanimously on it nearly a month ago, she thought it was brilliant. But now, revealing the catch phrase on the organization's swag for the first time, she wondered if the message would be clear. Hundreds of business cards and larger postcards also included the same question and QR code, and listed the same five principles of trauma-informed care. Feeling just a little anxious, Wendy sighed again and then got to work unloading their boxes and waiting for her other team members to arrive.

PLANNING WITHIN GRANT PARAMETERS

Wendy and Mae were at the breakfast networking event to represent the county change team, dubbed the trauma-informed, recovery-oriented system of care (TI-ROSC), for which Wendy was the official coordinator. The group had paid $250 from their TI-ROSC budget to the Chamber of Commerce to reserve one of the informational tables lining the back of the ballroom. Larger tables filled the center of the room, and those tables would soon be filled, within the hour, with business owners, executive directors, and otherwise active community members who were there to eat breakfast, network, and learn more about what local businesses and nonprofits were doing. Attendees could also visit one of two dozen or so tables at the back of the room, where local businesses and nonprofits provided more information about their products and services.

The TI-ROSC team was neither a business nor a nonprofit organization, but was a grant-funded workgroup under the newly formed local Addictions Coalition, which was supported by the university. The purpose of the TI-ROSC team was to infuse the community with more information about trauma-informed care, why it works and how to do it, specifically targeting professionals in their community that regularly interact with people misusing substances or in recovery from them.

The team came into being as a result of a one-year grant received by the local Addictions Coalition. The grant budget included a stipend to compensate a team coordinator, ideally a community member trained in group facilitation as well as trauma-informed care strategies. The organizers of the Addictions Coalition invited Wendy Radcliff to take on the role of TI-ROSC coordinator, and she accepted responsibility with enthusiasm. The budget also allowed for team members to be compensated with gift cards for the time spent in attendance at monthly meetings, and there was room in the budget to implement whatever change strategies the group decided upon, like paying to sponsor an informational table at the breakfast.

Wendy's first task as TI-ROSC coordinator was to determine the composition of the interdisciplinary team and invite community members to join. She recalled, "Deciding who to invite to the TI-ROSC team wasn't easy. There were so many talented, insightful, and knowledgeable community members who would have been excellent contributors, but with our budget, we could only afford to pay about 18 people per meeting. I also wanted the group to be representative of different neighborhoods, genders, ages, and races, so the task of composing the group felt nearly impossible. I did the best I could with recruitment, even though it wasn't perfect." She continued, "In the end, less than a dozen or people attended most meetings, so we had left over money in the budget where maybe I could have invited more."

Wendy's responsibilities as coordinator also meant she would facilitate all meetings, manage communication with members, oversee some type of community-wide needs assessment, and manage any initiatives that would emerge as a result of it.

Grant funding came from the state's Family and Social Service Administration, which had launched a TI-ROSC pilot project, led by the National Council for Behavioral Health, in two state counties three years earlier. The state's interest in supporting trauma-informed care came in response to the impact of the growing opioid epidemic in the state and decades of research evidence supporting the value of a trauma-informed approach when preventing or intervening in substance misuse.

As part of the original pilot project, the National Council worked closely with two counties within the state to develop a "tool kit" for implementing a TI-ROSC. The tool kit was organized into two sections. The first half presented concepts and data foundational to the effort, such as information about how and why a trauma-informed, recovery-oriented approach to care works, as well statistics on substance misuse in the state. The second half provided change tools that could be used to support the development of a county TI-ROSC. These tools were as follows:

- Readiness Checklist
- TI-ROSC Community Education Presentation
- Crafting a Compelling Story Tool
- Key Stakeholders List
- Trauma-Informed Care Principles Assessment Tool
- TI-ROSC Community Needs Assessment and Scoring Tools
- TI-ROSC Strengths, Weaknesses, Opportunities and Threats Assessment
- TI-ROSC Planning Tool 1: Visioning
- TI-ROSC Planning Tool 2: Necessary Components
- TI-ROSC Planning Tool 3: Components Sorting
- TI-ROSC Planning Tool 4: Action Planning
- TI-ROSC Strategic Plan Tracking Tool

Wendy led the TI-ROSC group's interdisciplinary members through several of the exercises provided in the tool kit during their regular monthly, three-hour meetings. In addition, the group crafted a mission and vision statement and administered a needs assessment survey to human services providers and stakeholders throughout the county. These stakeholders included people working in or receiving services from medical, behavior health, and criminal justice organizations as well as other social services related to housing, harm reduction, and community building. The TI-ROSC also included representatives from the library system and animal care and control, and people in recovery, many who were working as peer recovery coaches. Craig Boullion (see Chapter 10), an activist and street pastor in a neighborhood hard hit by the opioid crisis, was also part of the team.

After completing a survey-based community needs assessment and meeting to discuss short-term and long-term goals and strategies, the group decided to launch a trauma-informed care awareness campaign with two audiences in mind. The first audience would be the general public, and they would attempt to reach the public with advertisements in local mailers, as well as through tabling opportunities at community events.

"For three months, we took out an ad in a mailer called *Great Deals*," Wendy recalled. "We included our TI-ROSC catch phrase, 'Is your [blank] trauma-informed?' and the principles of trauma-informed care and the QR code leading back to a SAMHSA website about trauma-informed care. There's no way for us to know exactly how many people saw it, but several friends and coworkers told me they saw the ad."

The TI-ROSC wanted the public to gain an understanding of the role that trauma plays in substance misuse and recovery as a way to reduce shame and stigma. They also wanted the public to know that a trauma-informed, harm reduction approach to intervention was not only a compassionate approach but also one that was evidence-based and most likely to succeed. The group would set up their table with trauma-informed care information and swag at several events throughout the remainder of the year, including the Chamber of Commerce networking breakfast, in hopes to get the message out.

Mass media can often reach a larger audience than interpersonal efforts alone, yet there is an unrealistic assumption that mass media is an easy channel for creating widespread behavioral change. Knowledge alone is rarely enough to motivate behavior change. True cultural change is more complicated than merely injecting a message into a population.

When organizers send a message broadly into the community, it should be assumed that only some parts of the message will actually reach the intended target. The senders also cannot guarantee that the message will be received as intended.

Consistency of a message has been found to have the greatest impact. It is important to cast a wide net to reach as many people as consistently as possible (Green et al., 2015).

THE INTERSECTION OF SUBSTANCE USE DISORDER AND TRAUMA

Substance use disorder is a chronic but treatable disease where a person continues to misuse substances despite negative physical or social consequences, and effective intervention needs to address the root causes of the disorder. For many individuals, that root cause is related to trauma.

Trauma refers to acute (singular and sudden) or chronic (prolonged and anticipated) events that overwhelm a person's nervous system and ability to cope, temporarily and in the long term. People who experience acute or chronic trauma will often go into "fight or flight" mode, as their nervous system recognizes that their safety and well-being is at risk. Post-traumatic stress disorder (PTSD) occurs when the trauma has impacted the person's nervous system to the extent that even benign events may consciously or subconsciously remind them of the trauma, and their bodies will return to "fight or flight" mode even when the response is unnecessary (SAMHSA, 2014).

As a result of complex trauma, some people may have difficulty concentrating or relating to other people. They may feel numb and lack motivation, experiencing difficulty with executive functioning and decision making. They may experience intense irritability, anxiety, or paranoia. They may even feel unexplained physical pain in their bodies, a somatic reminder of the stress their minds have endured. Some may turn to addiction to mask the physical and emotional pain that they are feeling. For public health practitioners, clients who display these behaviors may be viewed erroneously as disengaged, noncompliant, lazy, and overall not worth helping (van Boekel et al., 2014).

What is trauma? **Trauma** refers to when a person's neurological capacity to cope with an event is overwhelmed.

Post-traumatic stress disorder (PTSD) can occur as a result of multiple types of trauma.

- *Acute trauma* (Type I trauma) results from one typically sudden and unexpected incident that is not likely to happen again, such as surviving a natural disaster or witnessing a homicide. Though every person responds differently to trauma, responses may include negative mood changes, intrusive memories, and avoidance of situations that trigger a memory of the event.

- *Chronic trauma* (Type II trauma) results from witnessing a series of events over time, such as prolonged exposure to community gun violence, that become repeated and anticipated. Responses to this type of trauma may be similar to those of acute trauma but also include dissociation, self-mutilation, and paranoia (Stefanovic et al., 2022).

- *Complex trauma* can result from chronic trauma that is severe and pervasive and often includes some type of physical or emotional captivity, such as in childhood abuse and neglect, domestic violence, organized sex trafficking, and living in a cult or concentration camp (Wamser-Nanney & Vandenberg, 2013).

Effective treatment for trauma includes relearning to regulate one's nervous system. Thus, the first step to healing from trauma is a living situation wherein the affected person can feel both physically and emotionally safe (SAMHSA, 2014).

Once safety has been reestablished, evidence-based treatment methods, such as eye movement desensitization and reprocessing (EMDR), exposure therapy (ET), cognitive processing therapy (CPT), and mindfulness-based stress reduction (MBSR) therapy can be helpful.

Decades of research has found a strong association between trauma and substance use disorders. People who experienced significant childhood trauma are at two to four times greater risk for early substance misuse and developing a substance use disorder. Moreover, people who misuse substances are also more likely to experience trauma, in part because they may be more likely to dissociate or less likely to accurately detect danger in their surroundings. This can lead to a harmful cycle where trauma increases risk of substance misuse, which then increases risk of exposure to more traumatic events, worsening substance misuse (**SAMHSA**, 2014).

Many adults have a mental illness, such as PTSD, depression, and/or anxiety, in addition to a substance use disorder. This condition is referred to as having a **co-occurring disorder**, and integrated treatment is recommended.

SAMHSA recommends that patients presenting with a mental health disorder should also be screened for a substance use disorder. Likewise, those presenting with a substance use disorder should be screened for mental health disorders (SAMHSA, 2020).

The notion of **trauma-informed care** in health services appears simple enough – when interacting with others, whether clients or coworkers, practitioners should proceed as if their clients and coworkers have a history of trauma, and avoid retraumatizing them. For many people with untreated trauma disorder, the body continues to store the memory of feeling unsafe and/or of feeling powerless to the point of danger. As such, re-traumatization can often occur when a person feels helpless or lacks control of their environment. For this reason, trauma-informed care typically includes components of choice, empowerment, and collaboration.

Wendy explained, "Trauma-informed care is good for overall community outcomes. If we want people impacted by substance use disorder to change their lifestyle and behavior, there must be must be safe physical and emotional spaces for them to do so."

She added, "Change isn't easy, even for people in peak health and wellness. And people rarely make good decisions when their body is constantly in a fight-or-flight state because of current or past reoccurring trauma."

One important characteristic of trauma-informed care is that, instead of asking "What's wrong with you?," practitioners might ask "What happened to you?"

Childhood trauma can be measured by a standard screening tool for **Adverse Childhood Experiences (ACEs)**. The questionnaire is comprised of 10 standard questions and used to measure potential trauma resulting from childhood.

Research has found that people who score a 4 or above on the ACEs screening are typically more at risk of a substance use disorder and other negative health and mental health consequences. However, protective factors, such as strong family support and participation in prosocial community activities, can mitigate the impact of ACEs. The questions are as follows:

Before the age of 18. . .

1. Did you feel that you did not have enough to eat, had to wear dirty clothes, or had no one to protect or take care of you?

2. Did you lose a parent through divorce, abandonment, death, or other reason?

3. Did you live with anyone who was depressed, mentally ill, or attempted suicide?

4. Did you live with anyone who had a problem with drinking or using drugs, including prescription drugs?

5. Did your parents or adults in your home ever hit, punch, beat, or threaten to harm each other?

6. Did you live with anyone who went to jail or prison?

7. Did a parent or adult in your home ever swear at you, insult you, or put you down?

8. Did a parent or adult in your home ever hit, beat, kick, or physically hurt you in any way?

9. Did you feel that no one in your family loved you or thought you were special?

10. Did you experience unwanted sexual contact (such as fondling or oral/anal/vaginal intercourse/penetration)?

STIGMA AS A BARRIER TO TRAUMA-INFORMED CARE

Based on their community needs assessment, the TI-ROSC team also identified helping professionals as an audience for information about trauma-informed care. Though a majority of professionals who completed the assessment indicated that they had heard of trauma-informed care or had at least one training in it, they admitted to needing more information for how to deliver it.

One essential task of a TI-ROSC county change team is to ensure that trauma-informed care is being delivered across a community's entire system of care for substance use disorders. To do so, a TI-ROSC team should complete a needs assessment to identify gaps in the continuum.

A **continuum of care** refers to an integrated system of care that guides and leads a person through all stages of healing and recovery. The continuum of care framework provided for the TI-ROSC team includes the following components (NCBH, 2023):

- Enhancing Health – Promoting physical and mental health and overall wellness, free from substance use disorders, with consistent health communication, income security, and access to services.

- Primary Prevention – Addressing individual and environmental risk factors for substance use disorders and strengthening protective factors, using evidence-based programs, policies, and strategies.

- Early Intervention – Screening for and detecting substance misuse at an early stage and providing brief intervention and other harm reduction activities.

- Treatment – Intervening through medication or counseling, such as provided by residential services and intensive outpatient programs (IOPs), to reduce symptoms and increase functional ability.

- Recovery Support – Providing long-term support and removing barriers to sobriety with the help of sober housing options as well as social, educational, mental, spiritual, and legal resources.

Wendy recruited another team member to help develop and facilitate an interactive one to two hour training for helping professionals, reiterating the connection between trauma and substance use disorder and the effective implementation of trauma-informed care. The interdisciplinary nature of the TI-ROSC team was helpful in helping in identifying groups that might need, and be receptive to, the training and connecting them with Wendy. As a result, the training was delivered to a variety of professionals, including foster care workers, medical residents, and social work students.

In some cases, our society practices trauma-informed care better with animals than humans.

Some veterinarian offices, for example, have become "fear-free certified" with the goal of reducing the anxiety and stress in pets during medical visits. They might implement a variety of strategies that create a setting of trauma-informed care, such as calming pheromone diffusers, tasty treats to act as distractions, heated blankets over cold slippery examination tables, and separate species-specific rooms. And, beyond simply implementing these practices, a trauma-informed veterinary clinic would commit to implementing a culture of trauma-informed care by only hiring staff who are similarly committed to administering fear-free services and use the same consideration toward all patients and each other.

These practices help not only the pets that attend these clinics, but also the veterinary practitioners who would work there because examining a furry patient, collecting blood samples, and administering shots and other medications is much easier when a pet is calm.

What does trauma-informed care look like with human beings? Many public health organizations struggle to define and deliver it. Stigma against people who struggle with substance use disorders presents a common barrier to creating a culture of trauma-informed care in an organization.

Stigma refers to stereotypical assumptions to all individuals within a group, a practice that devalues, dehumanizes, marginalizes, and isolates the group from social connection and opportunities that could otherwise be available to them (Corrigan & Kleinlein, 2005). An organization can attempt to implement trauma-informed education and practices in their service setting, but these strategies will fall flat if staff hold stigmatizing attitudes against people who misuse substances. Until fairly recently, substance misuse was often thought of as a moral failing rather than the chronic illness that it is. Unfortunately, people who experience stigma of any kind are less likely to seek help. Accordingly, the majority of people with substance use disorders in the US do not seek treatment, in part because of the stigma attached to it (Jones et al., 2020).

Research indicates that many healthcare professionals hold stigmatizing attitudes toward patients with substance abuse disorders, and this undermines the quality of care they provide. In one recent study, 75% of primary care physicians reported high levels of stigma toward people with substance use disorders (Gilchrist et al., 2011). Some healthcare practitioners do not engage with clients suspected of substance use disorders as they would with others, due to a belief that patients who abuse substances are irresponsible and unlikely to adhere to recommended treatment. Healthcare professionals might also misdiagnose patients who have substance use disorder by misattributing symptoms reported by patients (Puskar et al., 2013).

Moreover, some staff may come into the workplace with their own unresolved trauma around substance misuse, whether their own or someone's close to them, and their own fear, anxiety, and disappointment can be easily passed down or projected upon not only their clients but also other coworkers. In short, if a staff member is having difficulty addressing their own trauma, they may also struggle to address their client's trauma. In some cases, employees may simply need training for how to deliver trauma-informed care. But, as with many skills, there can be a gap between knowledge and behavior. And it will be more difficult for public health workers to deliver trauma-informed care if they are also dealing with their own trauma.

Healthcare professionals are in a unique position to identify substance use disorders and refer patients to treatment. However, many often receive limited training and may feel unprepared to work with this population, despite the prevalence of substance use disorders (Lindsay et al., 2017).

Research has found that healthcare professionals are most likely to engage with patients who are misusing substances when they have the following:

- Knowledge of how to appropriately engage, self-efficacy (role adequacy)
  Do they know what to do?
  Do they feel like they can make a difference?

- Belief that it is their responsibility to engage, and organizational policies/procedures support this belief (role legitimacy)
  Do they feel like it is their responsibility to engage/intervene with the patients' substance misuse?

- Belief that they will get support from their colleagues when engaging (role support)
  Will they have support/supervision while working with the patient?

HELPING THOSE WHO HELP

Making sense of substance use disorders is a difficult task. Friends and family members who help a loved one struggling might ask why the person continues to misuse substances despite negative consequences. It is not uncommon that they can become extremely frustrated when their help does not change the person's behavior. It can be difficult to understand why a person continues to use substances even though it hurts themselves and their loved ones. To someone who is not addicted, it simply does not make sense. But, at the core of substance use disorders, and an essential criterium for diagnosis, is that the person uses substances despite knowing that it undermines their best interests.

Helping professionals can also get frustrated when they see the see clients seemingly sabotage their health and success and continually return services. It is not uncommon for professionals who work with people struggling with substance misuse to experience professional burnout, as burnout is often associated with feeling ineffective in one's position (Holland et al., 2022). Moreover, helping professionals who work closely with this population can also experience vicarious or secondary trauma as a result of hearing about or witnessing another person's trauma. Learning a new trauma-informed approach to address substance use disorder can help professionals feel more impactful and can potentially help with their own trauma. The TI-ROSC was doing their part to get the message to the community: Is your _____ trauma informed?

DISCUSSION QUESTIONS

1. Discuss the pros and cons of various types of marketing "swag," including stickers, buttons, bracelets, T-shirts, stress balls, *Chap-Sticks*, and other types of items you may have encountered at resource fairs. Which swag items were most memorable or useful?

2. Discuss the difficulties of recruiting a small group of community members who are representative of various social service and public health sectors of the community as well as representative of different race/ethnicities, genders, income brackets, neighborhoods, ages, creeds, etc.

ACTIVITIES

1. Imagine that you are tasked with building an interdisciplinary county change team around a social need that impacts the entire community, but you can only invite a dozen people from various professional sectors to participate. Make a list of professionals you would invite and state why.

2. Do a web search for symptoms of a fight-or-flight response. Then, consider trying to make an important decision or complete a difficult task while experiencing these symptoms. In what ways might these symptoms hinder good decision-making or interfere with carrying out a detailed-oriented task? Discuss how holding down a job might be difficult while persistently in this state.

REFERENCES

Corrigan, P. W. & Kleinlein, P. (2005). *The Impact of Mental Illness Stigma*. Washington, DC: APA.

Gilchrist, C., Moskalewicz, J., Slezakova, S., Okruhlica, L., Torrens, M., Vajd, R., & Baldacchino, A. (2011). Staff regard toward working with substance users: A European multicentre study. *Addiction, 106*, 1114–1125.

Green, J., Tones, K., Cross, R., & Woodall, J. (2015). *Health Promotion: Planning & Strategies* (3rd ed.). Thousand Oaks, CA: Sage Publications.

Holland, M. L., Brock, S. E., Oren, T., & van Eckhardt, M. (2022). Introduction to Burnout and Trauma-Related Employment Stress. *Burnout and Trauma Related Employment Stress: Acceptance and Commitment Strategies in the Helping Professions* (pp. 1–16). New York: Springer Publishing.

Jones, C. M., Noonan, R. K., & Compton, W. M. (2020). Prevalence and correlates of ever having a substance use problem and substance use recovery status among adults in the United States, 2018. *Drug and Alcohol Dependence, 214*, 108–169. https://doi.org/10.1016/j.drugalcdep.2020.108169

Lindsay, D. L., Hagle, H., Lincoln, P., Williams, J., & Luongo, P. F. (2017). Exploring medical students' conceptions of substance use: A follow-up evaluation. *Substance Abuse, 38*(4), 464–467.

Puskar, K., Gotham, H. J., Terhorst, L., Hagle, H., Mitchell, A. M., Braxter, B., Fioravanti, M., Kane, I., Talcott, K. S., Woomer, G. R., & Burns, H. K. (2013). Effects of screening, brief intervention, and referral to treatment education and training on nursing students' attitudes toward working with patients who use alcohol and drugs. *Substance Abuse, 34*(2), 122–128.

Stefanovic, M., Ehring, T., Wittekind, C. E., Kleim, B., Rohde, J., Krüger-Gottschalk, A., Knaevelsrud, C., Rau, H., Schäfer, I., Schellong, J., Dyer, A., & Takano, K. (2022). Comparing PTSD symptom networks in type I vs. type II trauma survivors. *European Journal of Psychotraumatol, 13*(2). https://doi.org/10.1080/20008066.2022.2114260.

Substance Abuse and Mental Health Services Administration (2014). *SAMHSA's Concept of Trauma and Guidance for a Trauma-Informed Approach*. HHS Publication No. (SMA) 14-4884. Rockville, MD: Substance Abuse and Mental Health Services Administration.

Substance Abuse and Mental Health Services Administration. (2020). *Substance Use Disorder Treatment for People With Co-Occurring Disorders*. Treatment Improvement Protocol (TIP) Series, No. 42. SAMHSA Publication No. PEP20-02-01-004. Rockville, MD: Substance Abuse and Mental Health Services Administration.

The National Council for Behavioral Health for the Indiana Family and Social Service Administration (2023). *Trauma-informed Recovery-oriented Systems of Care Tool Kit*. https://www.thenationalcouncil.org/program/trauma-informed-recovery-oriented-systems-of-care-state-of-indiana/

van Boekel, L. C., Brouwers, E. P., van Weeghel, J., & Garretsen, H. F. (2014). Healthcare professionals' regard towards working with patients with substance use disorders: Comparison of primary care, general psychiatry and specialist addiction services. *Drug and Alcohol Dependence, 134*, 92–98.

Wamser-Nanney, R. & Vandenberg, B. R. (2013). Empirical support for the definition of a complex trauma event in children and adolescents. *Journal of Traumatic Stress, 26*, 671–678. https://doi.org/10.1002/jts.21857

CHAPTER

WORKING WITH EXTERNAL VENDORS

KNOWING WHAT TO LOOK FOR

In this special-focus chapter, we take you through the decision-making process of hiring an external vendor. In program planning, it is important to determine whether an organization has the in-house capacities to deliver a program or will need to hire an external vendor. Knowing the best practices for vetting and working with external vendors is useful.

Daveta Henry had a problem. She was the executive director of the local Court Appointed Special Advocate (CASA) program, a nonprofit organization dedicated to legal advocacy for children in the foster care system. Her role was to recruit, train, and supervise volunteers who would be CASAs for children involved in abuse and neglect cases. These volunteers would act as consistent support for the children, accompanying (or representing) them through multiple court hearings, foster placements, and a potentially high volume of case workers and clinicians. In the past quarter, Daveta had seen 400 more children than

Health Promotion Planning: Learning from the Accounts of Public Health Practitioners,
First Edition. Jean Marie S. Place, Jonel Thaller, and Scott S. Hall.
© 2024 John Wiley & Sons, Inc. Published 2024 by John Wiley & Sons, Inc.

average placed in the region's foster care system because of parental drug or alcohol addiction, and she lacked the needed CASA volunteers to be paired with these children. Worse, she knew that the flood of children entering the system was increasing, and it was largely attributable to the county's ever-growing opioid misuse problem.

This concern was shared by Judge O'Donnel and Magistrate Kennedy who both served in the county's juvenile court system. The question on their minds was how to stem the tide, or at least intervene, in parental drug and alcohol abuse early on so that the fallout did not affect children so severely. They were seeking a secondary prevention strategy – a way to detect early drug misuse and stop the problem from getting worse. In Daveta's daily interactions with the judges, along with law enforcement and sheriff's deputies, they talked about the importance of early detection of drug use and the need for education "to know what we're looking at and what we're looking for." This meant learning to "speak the language" of drug misuse in order to connect with the people who were active users and refer them to treatment, thereby preventing the downstream effects of child removals and an overburdened foster care system.

While attending a meeting, Daveta overheard the judges talking about someone called The Tall Cop. Standing at 6'9", Officer Jerome Galloway travels the country with a suitcase full of drug paraphernalia and a thumb drive full of slides to use as visual aids, training law enforcement, judges, educators, and community leaders to see drug references that are hiding in plain sight. During his well-attended presentations, Officer Galloway probes: Do you know what the sticker on that car means? The logo on that cap? Do you know how flavored drinks connect with music and drugs? He carefully tracks trends in popular culture, translating them so that professionals can read drug use references printed on clothing, ball caps, backpacks, and bottles. The Tall Cop wants to get the message out that the promotion of drugs is ubiquitous, though it may be flying just below the radar. Daveta heard about The Tall Cop and hoped he could help them increase their community's capacity to detect what was right before their eyes. The CASA program did not have sufficient knowledge about this topic to provide the education themselves.

Tall Cop Says Stop is a consulting company that "provides the tools, resources, and training to combat substance abuse."

Officer Galloway was recruited as external personnel, someone from outside an organization who fills a gap no one within the organization is able to do. The company *Tall Cop Says Stop* is referred to as an **external vendor** because it offers consulting and services at a price to organizations in need of health promotion programming.

Hiring Officer Galloway and flying him across the country from his home base in Boise, Idaho would cost several thousand dollars – no small cost for a nonprofit agency already operating on a tight budget. Daveta crafted a grant proposal that explained the need for an expert to train local professionals about emerging drug trends. When asked if a local sheriff could have stepped in to save costs and teach the same material, Daveta was sure she made the right move in hiring a vendor: "[Office Galloway's] knowledge is not just county-based, which is important... but he's also going to bring these trends to us that are maybe outside of what we know... We want to know what's out there, what's coming our way, what to look for, not just what we are already seeing. So, it was about bringing things we don't know to the people in our community."

SCREENING THE VENDOR

Daveta wanted to know that Office Galloway was selling a high-quality service, so she did a deep-dive into the testimonial section of the *Tall Cop Says Stop* website. She also reviewed the company's *Facebook* page and browsed the comments to see who his followers were. Comments like "I learned more in 1.5 hours than I have in 10 years!" propelled Daveta to pursue a contract. She commented, "I felt like I did my due diligence on making sure his product was high quality."

A section of the *Tall Cop Says Stop* website is devoted to Officer Galloway's credentials. For a man who played Division I basketball in college, his professional accomplishments are still listed like trading card stats: 105,000 people trained nationally and internationally; 60+ alcohol retail compliance checks; a conference that attracted 400 people from 28 states; 6 top awards and national recognitions; multiple instructor certifications; etc. The list goes on. It was enough to assure Daveta that she was dealing with someone who was qualified.

The quality of vendors varies. Program planners should note several considerations before selecting and entering into a contract with a vendor. Several key recommendations follow (McKenzie et al., 2017; Western Governors University, 2020):

▪ Noting things like whether the vendor was prepared, whether they listened to you, and their reputation can give you an idea about whether or not this is someone that you would like to work with.

- When hiring an external vendor, you want to make sure that the product or service they are offering is good quality. Openly sharing evidence of effectiveness is a good sign that a vendor has a quality product.

- It is always important to know whether a person is qualified to do the job you need them to do. Checking credentials can be a quick way to gauge a vendor's qualifications.

- Doing a bit of research on other vendors that provide a similar service can give you an idea of what that service usually costs. This can help you decide whether you think a vendor's price is fair for the service that they offer.

- A written contract is a great way to make sure both you and the vendor are on the same page when it comes to the service and how it is being delivered.

Daveta was a detail-oriented person. She noted how service was delivered in every interaction, with each positive encounter increasing her confidence that the grant funding would be well spent. Daveta recalled that, in her interactions with Officer Galloway or his small staff, she always felt they were in sync. Small details made her feel secure, like the way other staff members were cc'd on email responses and someone would always promptly follow up. Staff from *Tall Cop Says Stop* provided a written contract with a clause stipulating that no media be present during the presentation. She expressed appreciation in knowing these details upfront to avoid miscommunication and to help her agency plan the event.

The written contract specified that Daveta was to secure a suitable space to hold the workshop and obtain audiovisual equipment. An important question is whether a vendor has the technology equipment and skill to deliver the service. In Daveta's case, it was spelled out that Officer Galloway would bring the knowledge and expertise, but she needed to be in charge of the behind-the-scenes technology setup. Without clarification, these details could have been forgotten or overlooked. Daveta laughed to herself as she commented, "I tried hard to make sure technology needs were worked out ahead of time. Technology trouble would have been a nightmare on the day of the event!"

Other recommendations for working with external vendors include the following:

- Sorting out technology issues ahead of time can prevent potential disasters down the road. Having a plan for who is in charge of what will ensure that you have everything you need and that everything runs smoothly.

- Setting up a summative evaluation can help you determine whether the vendor met the needs of the audience, and whether a different approach might be better for the future.

EVALUATING THE WORK OF AN EXTERNAL VENDOR

Daveta took note of her initial impressions as she engaged with the vendor for the first time. She recalled being impressed with how Officer Galloway expressed concern about meeting the needs of her local community. She recounted her experience, "I told him who we were, why I was reaching out to him, the kinds of people that would be in our audience." With that information, he designed a session specific to our county. Rather than delivering a canned presentation, Officer Galloway makes each presentation highly class- and location-specific, lasting from one hour to two days, depending on need. As part of his process, he took a day prior to the workshop to do a community scan in the county, taking into account products sold at the shopping malls, smoke shops, and bars, and then weaving that needs assessment data into his formal presentation with ideas on how to combat the local drug culture.

To gauge the impact of the program, Daveta informally communicated with attendees during the two days of presentation. She asked them, "How's it going? How do you like it?" and recalled, "I don't think anybody said one negative thing about it." Daveta relied on informal conversation and observation to learn whether the training was helpful. Officer Galloway likely received positive comments from satisfied attendees, but no survey-based, summative evaluation took place at the conclusion of the event to measure people's satisfaction with what they had seen, heard, and learned.

Daveta had not shopped around for other vendors – she knew that she wanted to bring in The Tall Cop from the moment she overheard Judge O'Donnel and Magistrate Kennedy talking about him. Moreover, because Officer Galloway's service was so unique, it may have been difficult to compare his cost and value to that of other vendors. In total, the cost of bringing The Tall Cop to the county was $7290, which included travel and accommodation, as well as providing two breakfasts, two lunches, and space and equipment rental. This amounted to roughly $50 per person per day when divided by the 75 people who attended the two-day training. Daveta commented, "I'm thinking that's actually not bad at all."

DISCUSSION QUESTIONS

1. How could you assess the impact of external personnel on a target population?

2. How could you conduct a formative evaluation on "product quality"?

3. How important is anecdotal evidence? How much weight should it have compared to other sources?

ACTIVITY

1. Compare and contrast benefits and disadvantages of utilizing internal versus external personnel for services, programs, and expertise.

REFERENCES

McKenzie, J., Neiger, B., & Thackeray, R. (2017). *Planning, Implementing, and Evaluating Health Promotion Programs: A Primer*. USA: Pearson.

Western Governors University (2020). How to Manage Vendors Effectively. https://www.wgu.edu/blog/how-to-manage-vendors-effectively2008.html#close

CHAPTER

13

WORKING WITH VOLUNTEERS

LEARNING MANAGEMENT SKILLS

In this special-focus chapter, we showcase a volunteer coordinator who is skilled at recruiting and managing a range of volunteers in a domestic violence shelter. Volunteers are an important human resource that can be leveraged for the success of health promotion programs.

The once-grand, nineteenth century Victorian home stood out from the rest of the ho-hum brick dwellings on the street. Intricate woodwork lined the front porch like lace, so dainty and beautiful that it was easy to overlook the lavender and white paint peeling from it. Little did most people know that this home was functioning as a domestic violence shelter with a robust, rotating set of volunteers who helped staff the shelter, as well as an accompanying suicide hotline. Stepping through the covered porch, Anna, a middle-aged woman and faithful volunteer, rang the bell and waited to be buzzed in. Inside was warm and colorful. Behind the front desk, opposite from the white banister,

Health Promotion Planning: Learning from the Accounts of Public Health Practitioners, First Edition. Jean Marie S. Place, Jonel Thaller, and Scott S. Hall.
© 2024 John Wiley & Sons, Inc. Published 2024 by John Wiley & Sons, Inc.

there was a small room with muted voices offering reassurance over the clicking of fingers on computer keys. It was the room hosting the suicide resource hotline with volunteers fielding calls from around the nation. Other female voices whirred, and as the door clicked shut, a pair of staff nodded her way – a quick swivel to greet her and then a near-simultaneous pivot back to the conversation. The message was clear: anyone who wanted to contribute was welcome to step in, roll up their sleeves, and get to work.

Staff at domestic violence shelters often interface with women who use substances. At this shelter, women are not allowed to use substances on the premises although off-site use is permitted. When use is detected, women are referred to inpatient or outpatient substance use services.

Suicide, domestic violence, and substance use are often connected. Each can be influenced by the same problems, such as poverty and mental illness, and each can also contribute to the occurrence of one another. When someone has two or more medical conditions, each condition is considered a **comorbidity** – a condition that coexists with another condition. Similarly, people often struggle with multiple challenges at the same time.

Anyone who is experiencing domestic violence, sexual assault, thoughts of suicide, depression, loneliness, substance misuse, or just needs someone to talk to can call 765-288-HELP or 988. In partnership with the National Suicide Prevention Lifeline, this hotline has been accredited by Contact USA and connects callers with the best advice and resources available for their situation.

Anna was one of the approximately 50 volunteers the organization integrated every six months. The number of volunteers rotating into the shelter was significantly more than in the past and regularly exceeded the 40 full- and part-time paid employees serving the 20-bed shelter. Many of these volunteers were busy stripping beds, helping children with their homework, and chopping vegetables for nightly meals. Others were working in the walk-in rape crisis center, facilitating substance use support groups, and staffing phones for the 24-hour crisis line, suicide hotline, and check-in call service for elderly and disabled homebound people. Anna maintained the donation room in tip-top order, as well as coordinating the secondhand clothes and appliances that filtered in from garage sales and spring cleaning. A few years prior, there was a shortage of personal care items used by the residents due to a funding problem; federal dollars had been allocated to the shelter but the state was behind in rolling assistance out across the region, so they had not yet received their funding allotment. A *Facebook* request was posted asking for donations, and the plug generated a community-wide out-pouring of toilet paper and toiletries. Anna ended up organizing this massive influx of deodorants, shampoos, and toothpaste.

Program planning can incorporate identifying, recruiting, selecting, and training volunteers, particularly if an agency lacks sufficient staff or has limited financial resources. Research has shown that volunteers can effectively step in to lead or assist with program implementation, expanding the program's reach beyond what would be possible with paid staff only (Substance Abuse and Mental Health Services Administration [SAMHSA, n.d.]).

Creating a job description for prospective volunteers, including position title, duties, required qualifications, and desired experience is helpful guidance for everyone involved. Because many volunteers end up taking on roles that paid employees would otherwise do, volunteers should be evaluated just as a prospective employee would be.

COORDINATING VOLUNTEER EFFORTS

Shayna Fellows, a happy woman with short, spiky gray hair and a soothing low voice, is the shelter's volunteer coordinator. She recruited and managed the revolving door of volunteers, which required great effort, planning, and organization to make the most of the help. Shayna explained the variety of ways volunteers like Anna ended up coming to the shelter to provide volunteer hours. She outlined the steps: To start, Shayna sits down and interviews potential volunteers, listening carefully and kindly about their motivation for volunteering. Shayna listens for a crucial key to success, that the volunteer's orientation toward clients reflects the organization's philosophy. Is it consistent? Do they have a heart for empowering marginalized men and women? She also needs to match a person's skills and desires to specific oppor-tunities for service. Some volunteers may want time to themselves. If so, they are good candidates for the donation room. Others want to interact with clients. She corrected herself, "need to *learn how* to interact with clients." She puts them with groups of women and kids who are milling around common spaces before dinner where volunteers can play games, chat up teenagers, or read to the preschoolers and kindergarteners, some of whom will not speak at all due to the pro-found trauma from their recent upheaval.

The shelter also hosts a Monday night support group at a neighboring church. Graduate student interns lead the discussion while nonclinical volunteers provide childcare, prepare dinner, and circle up chairs for the clients' group therapy sessions. Shayna tries to let volunteers give input on where and how to spend their time, though she puts some parameters around their involvement: At least three hours a week should be spent volunteering at the shelter. She even requires students who may only need to complete 25 volunteer hours to stay for a whole semester. "It is a lesson in not quitting," she emphasized.

It is important to determine if volunteers will serve in (1) direct care positions (interacting with clients), (2) indirect service positions (carry out services behind the scenes without direct contact with clients), (3) internal administrative roles (such as secretarial work), or (4) external administrative roles (such as fundraising or public relations).

Best practices for using volunteers include giving them autonomy about where and how to spend their time (Bidee et al., 2013). Giving people choice and encouragement for personal initiative and competence is associated with less volunteer turnover (Gagne, 2003) and higher volunteer satisfaction (Oostlander et al., 2014).

VolunteerMatch.com is a useful online site to help potential volunteers find service opportunities that match interests.

Shayna had considered various ways to recruit long-term volunteers, hoping to rely less on the transience of a student population and more on community volunteers. She reached out to parishioners and congregants of faith-based institutions, as well as other baby boomers, but found it hard to recruit in those sectors compared to the usefulness of colleges and universities who can make community service part of graduation requirements. Still, even in the age of social media and mass media outlets, one-on-one conversations and word-of-mouth invitations remained her most effective method, particularly if she spoke at an outreach event where the audience felt informed, educated, and energized.

Because many of the volunteers are undergraduate and graduate students from the local university, Shayna made note of some unique elements of working with student volunteers. She said that college students can be motivated to volunteer to gain work-related experience, build a resume, and develop professional skills. While many students are there to complete service hours required by a psychology, health science, or social work course, other students show up because they are go-getters who are inspired by the organization's mission and signed up through Student Volunteer Services or approached the shelter's booth at volunteer fairs.

Shayna related a story of two medical school residents who volunteered at the shelter without any outside entity counting their hours or incentivizing their involvement. They were motivated by a desire to learn more about low-resourced women's lived experiences so they could better provide healthcare services that holistically address them. One paid staff member began as an unpaid volunteer, getting her foot in the door of an organization whose mission she believed in. Shayna talked about volunteers who show up because they want to "give back" or "have a purpose to get up each morning." Shayna commented, "You want someone whose heart is really in it, though motives alone do not make for an effective volunteer."

Researchers report volunteers want to stay active, have social interaction, and use gifts and talents (Van Der Wagen & Carlos, 2005). It is important to understand the intrinsic or external motivations of volunteers so coordinators can place individuals in roles that suit them and thus have a higher chance of retaining them, which is critical given the investment required to train them.

For example, older and young adults tend to perceive the benefits of volunteering differently, likely as a result of their differing motives for involvement. When volunteering, older adults perceive greater increases in life satisfaction over time as well as greater perceived changes in health (Van Willigen, 2000).

TRAINING VOLUNTEERS

All volunteers at the shelter undergo an eight-hour training, all in one day, either on a Wednesday or a Saturday. Shayna mentioned that four trainings with volunteers had already been held the past two months. Many volunteers sit next to new employees as part of their onboarding process – a testament to volunteers being equal shareholders in conducting the daily activities of the shelter and upholding the organization's mission and values. Three of the eight hours are dedicated to training all volunteers on the suicide hotline. Volunteers take turns staffing the hotline where people call in about their crises, but not before their comfort level grows through observation and listening in on different calls.

For some agencies, training volunteers can be a burden, requiring more time and effort than they have to spare. An innovative solution to this challenge is to work collaboratively with other organizations to create one community-wide volunteer training that addresses basic concepts common to many social service and health organizations, including absenteeism, use of agency resources (such as copiers), expenses and reimbursement, liability, and conflict resolution (Schneider et al., 2007).

Older, religious adults in good health with higher income and more education typically volunteer more often than their counterparts (Urban Institute, 2006). Those who volunteer are also likely to be married to a spouse who volunteers. To recruit retirees, involve them in agency activities while they are still in the workforce.

Most volunteers need to be supervised and periodically evaluated. Shayna provides each volunteer with a 40-page packet that includes background information on the organization, confidentiality agreements, and dress code requirements. She monitors volunteer hours by having individuals check in and out on a log near the front desk. She does not have the time to shadow volunteers, especially students, but she occasionally checks in with coworkers who interact more directly with the volunteer to see how they are doing. She will provide grades for students at the behest of professors and preceptors on a one-to-five scale at midterm and finals, but mostly her office is open for volunteers to come in informally and discuss issues and request support.

It is important to recognize volunteers' efforts in staff meetings, at appreciation ceremonies, or in newsletters, news releases, and other public venues.

Recognition is a key to retention, along with providing training, professional development, and appropriately matching skill sets with organizational tasks (Cho et al., 2020). On the opposite end of the spectrum, organizations are encouraged to "express opinions about poor volunteer performance in a diplomatic way" (Van Der Wagen & Carlos, 2005, p. 180) and to let poor performers go.

Shayna has been known to take volunteers out for lunch to say thank you. She can only really recall two problematic volunteers who tried to log hours without completing them. However, when termination needs to occur or volunteers resign, Shayna found that conducting exit interviews can lead to helpful feedback to improve the volunteer experience for the future. Shayna chuckled as she reflected on the many volunteers whom she has supervised. When it is time to say goodbye, she said, usually it is nothing but hugs, kisses, and tears.

DISCUSSION QUESTIONS

1. What components of working with volunteers are important for program planners to consider while in the planning process? What might make it challenging to do so?

2. What are some ways you could bolster recruitment of volunteers to serve in an agency?

3. What are ways that a volunteer coordinator could increase a sense of autonomy among volunteers?

4. Have you been a formal volunteer at an organization? Describe your internal motivation for doing so. What was your external motivation?

ACTIVITY

1. Read the following peer-reviewed article and identify questions you have about the material. Provide a verbal summary of the article in class.

   Bird, Y., Islam, A., and Moraros, J. (2016). Community-based clinic volunteering: An evaluation of the direct and indirect effects on the experience of health science college students. *BMC Medical Education, 16*, 21. https://www.ncbi.nlm.nih.gov/pmc/articles/PMC4717538/pdf/12909_2016_Article_547.pdf.

REFERENCES

Bidee, J., Vantilborgh, T., Pepermans, R., & Willems, J. (2013). Autonomous motivation stimulates volunteers' work effort: A self-determination theory approach to volunteerism, *International Journal of Voluntary and Nonprofit Organizations, 24*, 32–47.

Cho, H., Wong, Z., & Chiu, W. (2020). The effect of volunteer management on intention to continue volunteering: A mediating role of job satisfaction of volunteers. *Sage Open.* https://doi.org/10.1177/2158244020920588.

Gagné, M. (2003). The role of autonomy support and autonomy orientation in prosocial behavior engagement. *Motivation and Emotion, 27*(3), 199–223. https://doi.org/10.1023/A:1025007614869

Oostlander, J., Guntert, S., Van Schie, S., & Wehner, T. (2014). Leadership and volunteer motivation: A study using self-determination theory. *Nonprofit and Voluntary Sector Quarterly, 43*(5), 869–889.

Schneider, E., Altpeter, M., Whitelaw, N. (2007). *An innovative approach for building health promotion capacity: A generic volunteer training curriculum. The Gerontologist, 47(3),* 398–403.

Substance Abuse and Mental Health Services Administration (n.d.). Successful strategies for recruiting, training and utilizing volunteers. https://www.samhsa.gov/sites/default/files/volunteer_handbook.pdf

Urban Institute (2006). *Older Adults Engaged as Volunteers.* https://www.urban.org/research/publication/older-adults-engaged-volunteers

Van Der Wagen, L. & Carlos, B. (2005). *Event Management: For Tourism, Cultural, Business, and Sporting Events.* Upper Saddle River, NJ: Pearson Prentice Hall.

Van Willigen, M. (2000). Differential benefits of volunteering across the life course. *The Journals of Gerentology, 55*(5), S308–S318.

CHAPTER

14

WORKING ACROSS INSTITUTIONS

SHARING KNOWLEDGE ON SUBSTANCE USE DISORDERS

In this special-focus chapter, we learn from the account of a local team that joined a state-wide network to exchange information about substance use disorder programming. In program planning, it is important to use appropriate, up-to-date language to describe the health problem, understand treatment options, and confront social stigma.

BUILDING STRONG, PERSON-CENTERED RELATIONSHIPS

The small, square conference room at the local Coordinating Council Substance Use Prevention (CCSUP) office had been transformed. A large projection screen covered the wall where a whiteboard usually appeared. Darby Montegro, executive director, mumbled while trying to adjust the laptop and projector on a table in the center of the room,

Health Promotion Planning: Learning from the Accounts of Public Health Practitioners,
First Edition. Jean Marie S. Place, Jonel Thaller, and Scott S. Hall.
© 2024 John Wiley & Sons, Inc. Published 2024 by John Wiley & Sons, Inc.

which was encircled by tables and chairs set up for members of the newly formed team. There was significant nervous energy among the dozen attendees, with many people wondering aloud what was going to happen in this first meeting. A cluster of attendees were discussing what SPOKE might stand for – the name the newly formed team had been given – assuming it was an acronym. Darby explained that it was meant as an analogy, that counties across the state are like spokes of a wheel, and the purpose of the meeting was for counties to learn from one another about substance use disorder recovery efforts.

The words we use to describe substance use and people who struggle with substance use disorders affect our perceptions and attitudes toward people.

"Substance use disorder" is a contemporary way to describe what in the past might have been called "drug abuse." While older terminology is still heard today, especially in casual conversation among the general public, many professionals and advocates who work with people who have substance use related disorders argue for the use of precise, person-first language (NIDA, 2023).

For example, *abuse* has a more negative, judgmental tone than *use* (for illicit drugs) and *misuse* (often describing prescription medication being used other than as prescribed). Negative, judgmental attitudes can contribute to shame, which can reinforce substance use.

Describing the compulsion to use substances as a disorder is preferred to describing people as choosing to do drugs. The connotations of having a disorder – an illness – arguably create more empathy and compassion and less judgment of someone struggling with substance misuse.

Using the term "disorder" is a way to emphasize that substance misuse reaches a point at which it is beyond a person's control to stop using the substance, or that stopping it without professional intervention could be dangerous. This is in contrast to the misinformed notion that substance misuse is a moral failing.

Consider how these proposed word changes (Ashford et al., 2019) influence how we think about these issues: Instead of "relapsed" say "had a setback," and instead of "stayed clean" say "maintained recovery."

The SPOKE team was assembled in response to the state's Department of Health that had been awarded a grant from the Centers for Disease Control and Prevention (CDC) to do the following:

- increase comprehensiveness and timeliness of drug overdose surveillance data
- the Prescription Drug Monitoring Program more user-friendly

- work with health systems, insurers, and communities to improve opioid prescribing and
- build state and local capacity for public health programs related to substance use disorder

As part of this grant, the Department of Health invited counties throughout the state to apply to be part of the newly formed Extension for Community Healthcare Outcomes (ECHO) project. In short, ECHO was a way to organize communication among the different counties involved in this effort, with the counties being like the spokes of a wheel (like the director had explained), and a hub team (center of the wheel) acting as the centralized organizers of the collaboration. The local county SPOKE team received funding from the Department of Health to help support their involvement.

The team members around the room briefly introduced themselves while waiting for the virtual broadcast to begin. They represented various sectors in the county, including law enforcement, medical establishments, drug treatment programs, social services, and the local university. The grant required that at least five different sectors be represented on each team. Suddenly a multitude of additional faces appeared on the screen as the voice of the host echoed through the speakers. The hub team, broadcasting from a large metropolitan area, introduced themselves and gave a brief overview of the agenda. A dozen or so counties were represented in the videoconference, mostly with teams grouped in conference rooms. A friendly face instructed everyone to introduce themselves, one person at a time, after the name of each county was mentioned. With upwards of 100 people involved, some faces seemed to grimace about the questionable use of time.

While building connections among team members is important, it seemed doubtful that a long string of three-second introductions would have the desired effect. Creating a sense of unity and trust for a state-wide group this large would be very difficult. The local team sitting in the same room would likely have more success forming a unified team, though as of yet no time had been allotted for doing so.

Ideally, when forming a team, team members should share a passion for their joint purposes, and members should feel free to share their perspectives with the confidence that they will be heard and respected. Establishing this kind of rapport among team members is sometimes referred to as a process of "forming" (Butterfoss, 2007). A key part of forming is understanding the purposes and logistics of operation, like how the meetings would roll out and the typical procedures, which help people know what to expect. Investing in some time up front to help team members feel comfortable with another, to understand everyone's motivations and expertise, and to know procedural expectations can help foster more productive discussions and teamwork in later meetings.

Common steps of team development, in addition to "forming," include "storming" (working through differences of opinion on determining goals, roles, and procedures), "norming" (solidifying roles and relationships, establishing interdependence), "performing" (working toward team goals, further delegation of tasks), and "reforming" (team may continue but refocus efforts on other tasks). At some point, most teams disband after completing their goals or due to lack of effectiveness. Some team members have been known to then enter into a phase of "mourning" (Butterfoss, 2007), given that people might miss being part of a team.

After introductions, the main facilitator described the format for this and subsequent meetings and the roles that various participants would play. Each meeting would include one or more formal presentations related to substance use. After the presentations, a team from one of the counties would share a case study, describing a specific challenge they faced while addressing substance use disorder issues. General expectations for language use were also explained, namely, using person-first language was encouraged.

Person-first language, similar to the preferred ways of describing substance misuse mentioned earlier, is another way to reduce stigma associated with SUD. For example, say "a person with a substance use disorder," "a person with an addiction," or "a person in recovery" instead of referring to someone as an "addict," "druggie," or "junkie." Similarly, think about the difference between calling someone an "ex-addict" vs "a person living in recovery" (Ashford et al., 2019).

Research supports the idea that people do better in recovery when attitudes toward addiction are less negative and judgmental (Kennedy-Hendricks et al., 2017). The words we use – including how people with substance disorders describe themselves – can amplify or neutralize counterproductive perceptions of people.

From a program planning standpoint, deliberate word choices are important for messaging about the purposes and outcomes of your program and the population you hope to help.

For this first meeting, a presenter from the CDC shared national overdose trends, followed by a presenter from a state-based agency who spoke about statewide overdose trends and medication-assisted treatment (MAT). The discussion also centered on roadblocks to treatment, especially to the use of MAT in the prisons. Much was said about public and institutional stigma surrounding MAT. The meeting concluded with a discussion that included clarifying questions (seeking additional information about the case) and recommendations. This was the main purpose of the meeting after all, to draw from the expertise and experiences of individuals, teams, and agencies across the state to help solve local substance related problems. It was encouraging to hear from a handful of counties who had made strides toward reducing the stigma of using MAT through community education efforts.

Medication-assisted treatment (MAT) is "the use of medications in combination with counseling and behavioral therapies, which is effective in the treatment of opioid use disorders (OUDs) and can help some people to sustain recovery" (US Food & Drug Administration, 2023). Three medications have been approved for this purpose and have been shown to be safe and effective when used in combination with psychosocial support and counseling: buprenorphine, methadone, and naltrexone.

These medications help to minimize cravings for addictive substances, and buprenorphine and methadone can also treat withdrawal symptoms. When used correctly, these medications do not produce a "high."

Individual treatment plans are created and closely monitored. The length of time for MAT depends on the individual and the success of one's social and emotional support network. Methodone is administered orally within treatment programs that require daily visits to certified clinics. Buprenorphine and naltrexone must be prescribed by a qualified professional. Buprenorphine can be ingested orally (under the tongue or in the cheek), injected, or implanted, and naltrexone can be taken orally or be injected.

MAT is still catching on among clinicians, though a lack of sufficient knowledge and training limits its accessibility. Stigmatized attitudes among the public can also slow the adoption of MAT throughout the country.

Before signing off, the facilitator previewed next month's meeting, including the date and time (another important part of the *forming* stage of team building). People in the room quickly grabbed their jackets and headed toward the exit, presumably to get back to their various places of employment. By the end, the meeting format and ultimate purpose for having SPOKE teams had become clear.

FIGHTING STIGMA AS A PART OF PROGRAM PLANNING

During the COVID-19 pandemic, subsequent SPOKE meetings happened completely virtually. Instead of local teams meeting together to engage with the virtual broadcast, individuals logged in from their own particular locations. Fortunately, the second meeting was run more efficiently – verbal introductions were limited to the hub team while everyone else typed their names and respective counties into a chat box. The facilitator asked that screen names include affiliations and for everyone to turn on their cameras to promote more personal connections. Most complied, and seeing a baby or two appear in the backgrounds was a bonus. The format of the meeting was otherwise the same – formal presentations about a SUD related topic, then a case study presented by a specific county seeking and receiving broad input on how to face their particular challenges. These challenges were often related to attitudes and awareness within the general community.

One such community challenge that was mentioned multiple times each meeting was the problem of social **stigma** – negative attitudes associated with long-term recovery treatments (e.g. MAT), HIV testing, needle exchange programs, and addiction in general. Such stigma was argued to inhibit people from seeking treatment and to overly restrict the types of treatments that communities could offer. In this case, some community-level leaders and practitioners had concerns about certain types of interventions and programs (e.g. needle exchange) and would use their influence to prevent them from being implemented in their county. Other individuals likely personally supported the interventions and programs but felt pressure from the broader community to oppose their implementation.

When resistance to programming is driven by stigma, misinformation, and stereotypes about people with SUDs, program planners should consider dedicating time and other resources toward helping transform a community into a more health-enhancing environment (Hunnicutt & Leffelman, 2006). Specifically, procedures may need to be implemented that educate a community or general public about the usefulness and necessity of certain activities or interventions and challenge outdated assumptions and beliefs.

Proceed with caution when using such approaches to avoid coming across as dismissive of diverse perspectives, however. Changing hearts and minds can take time and usually requires a genuine, personal connection with caring and well-informed individuals.

Most of the ECHO meetings included breakout sessions in which small groups discussed the presented information. In one breakout session, the local SPOKE team discussed the available county-based services for their clients and how service providers rely on the local YMCA and other organizations to help advertise such services. They concluded that resources were lacking, especially for men, and that creating recovery residencies that allow individuals to connect with local MAT providers could be beneficial.

At the conclusion of a year of monthly meetings, county SPOKE teams were asked to discuss and document the benefits they observed from participating in these ECHO sessions. Feedback was gathered and sent to the Department of Health where it was aggregated and then sent out to all SPOKE teams for their review. Ultimately, it was up to each county to plan and implement any changes that were inspired by these informational exchanges with their contemporaries across the state.

DISCUSSION QUESTIONS

1. What value can come from making personal connections with other team members or community collaborators?

2. What helps you feel connected to people you do not know?

3. Have you ever been labeled in a way that would make you feel resentful and less likely to receive someone's offer to help?

4. Have you ever had someone change your mind about a controversial topic? What made the effort to change your mind successful?

5. How can you anticipate attitudes in the community that might hamper your efforts to reach your target population? How can you plan for confronting those attitudes?

ACTIVITY

1. Using what you learned about preferred word choices and about medically-assisted treatment (MAT), craft a letter to the

state governor the explains the importance of considering more treatment options for people with opioid use disorder (OUD) and with recommendations on how to reduce stigma in the community toward OUD (including why it is important to reduce stigma).

REFERENCES

Ashford, R. D., Brown, A., & Curtis, B. (2019). Expanding language choices to reduce stigma: A Delphi study of positive and negative terms in substance use and recovery. Health Education, *119*(1), 51–62. https://doi.org/10.1108/HE-03-2018-0017

Butterfoss, F. D. (2007). *Coalitions and Partnerships in Community Health*. San Francisco, CA: Jossey-Bass.

Hunnicutt, D., & Leffelman, G. (2006). WELCOA's 7 benchmarks of success. *Absolute Advantage, 6*, 2–29.

Kennedy-Hendricks, A., Barry, C. L., Gollust, S. E., Ensminger, M. E., Chisolm, M. S., & McGinty, E. E. (2017). Social stigma toward persons with prescription opioid use disorder: Associations with public support for punitive and public health–oriented policies. Psychiatric Services, *68*(5), 462–469. https://doi.org/10.1176/appi.ps.201600056

National Institute of Drug Addiction (2023, June 23). *Words Matter: Preferred Language for Talking About Addiction.* https://nida.nih.gov/research-topics/addiction-science/words-matter-preferred-language-talking-about-addiction

U.S. Food & Drug Administration (2023, May 23). *Information about Medication-Assisted Treatment (MAT).* https://www.fda.gov/drugs/information-drug-class/information-about-medication-assisted-treatment-mat

INDEX

Note: "b" = appears only in grey textbox on that page.